CLINICIANS IN COURT

Clinicians in Court

*A Guide to Subpoenas, Depositions,
Testifying, and Everything Else
You Need to Know*

ALLAN E. BARSKY
JONATHAN W. GOULD

THE GUILFORD PRESS
New York   London

© 2002 The Guilford Press
A Division of Guilford Publications, Inc.
72 Spring Street, New York, NY 10012
www.guilford.com

Printed in the United States of America

This book is printed on acid-free paper.

Last digit is print number: 9 8 7 6 5 4 3 2 1

Library of Congress Cataloging-in-Publication Data

Barsky, Allan Edward.
    Clinicians in court : a guide to subpoenas, depositions, testifying,
and everything else you need to know / Allan E. Barsky, Jonathan W.
Gould.
        p. cm.
Includes bibliographical references and index.
Derived from a Canadian version titled Counsellors as witnesses,
published by Canada Law Book in 1997.
    ISBN 1-57230-788-9 (acid-free paper)
  1. Evidence, Expert—United States.   2. Witnesses—United States.   3.
Clinics—Employees—Legal status, laws, etc.—United States.   I. Gould,
Jonathan W., 1953-   II. Barsky, Allan Edward. Counsellors as witnesses.
III. Title.
KF8961 .B37 2002
347.73'67—dc21
                                                        2002007880

About the Authors

Allan E. Barsky, JD, MSW, PhD, is Professor of Social Work at Florida Atlantic University in Boca Raton, where he teaches graduate courses in conflict resolution, professional ethics, and substance abuse. Dr. Barsky received his JD from the University of Toronto (1983), his MSW from Yeshiva University in New York City (1988), and his PhD from the University of Toronto (1995). Dr. Barsky has practiced social work and mediation in legal settings that include the criminal court in New York and the family courts in New York, Toronto, and Ft. Lauderdale. He is a past president of the Ontario Association for Family Mediation and former National Board Member of the Network for Conflict Resolution Canada. His book credits include *Conflict Resolution for the Helping Professions* (Brooks/Cole, 2000), *Interprofessional Practice with Diverse Populations* (Greenwood, 2000), and *Counsellors as Witnesses* (Canada Law Book, 1997). His research has been published in *Family and Conciliation Courts Review, Mediation Quarterly, Negotiation Journal,* and *Revista de Treball Social* (Spain). His research has also been presented at international conferences in Helsinki, Amsterdam, Jerusalem, and Hong Kong.

Jonathan W. Gould, PhD, is in private practice in Charlotte, North Carolina, where he is a principal in the Charlotte Psychotherapy and Consultation Group. He obtained his BS in psychology from Union College (1975), his MA and CAS in school psychology from SUNY, College at Plattsburgh (1978), and his PhD in counseling psychology from SUNY at Albany (1985). He also completed a year of specialized training in marriage, family, and sex therapy at the Marriage Council of Philadelphia at the University of Pennsylvania (1984). His book credits include *Reinventing Fatherhood* (TAB/McGraw-Hill, 1993) and *Conducting Scientifically Crafted Child Custody Evaluations* (Sage, 1998). His works have appeared in *Family and Conciliation Courts Review, Family Court Review, Professional Psychology: Research and Practice*, and *Juvenile and Family Court Journal*. Dr. Gould's interests focus on developing more scientific approaches to child custody evaluations, defining role boundaries between clinical and forensic treatment, and applying forensic methods and procedures to child custody evaluations. He has presented workshops or seminars for the American Psychological Association, the Association of Family and Conciliation Courts, the National Council of Juvenile and Family Court Judges, the Family Law section of the American Bar Association, the North Carolina Academy of Trial Lawyers, and the California Administrative Offices of the Court.

Preface

The contents of this book are for information purposes only and should not be construed as providing legal advice. Laws vary widely among the states, and the only certainty in law is that laws will change. Although the suggestions in this book may assist you in handling a specific situation, your only true protection may require obtaining independent legal advice from a properly licensed attorney[1] who specializes in the areas of law that are relevant to your case. We disclaim all legal liability for reliance on this material.

"Arrrgh! Not another disclaimer—and in fine print, no less. Can't I get a straight answer out of these attorneys? They make everything so complicated. Do they always have to cover their behinds?"
We confess. Law is complicated. Easy answers are possible. However, easy answers are possibly misleading. We don't want to expose ourselves to lawsuits, but we also don't want to mislead or expose you to legal liabilities. With all of these disclaimers, what good is this book? You can use this book for a number of purposes:

- To gain general professional knowledge.
- To know how to inform clients about many of the legal implica-

---

[1]One of the advantages of retaining the services of a licensed attorney is that the attorney will have liability insurance to cover any damages you incur that arise from negligent errors or omissions by the attorney. For cases involving clinicians, the most relevant areas of law are generally mental health law, criminal law, family law, human rights, and professional malpractice.

tions of their professional therapeutic relationship (e.g., a client who wants to talk to you in confidence, or a client who is asking you to assess and provide an opinion or recommendation).

- To prepare for or avoid situations in which you might be called to testify as an expert or nonexpert witness.
- To prepare for a particular court action or adjudicative proceeding when you have been called to testify.
- To devise strategies to deal with emotional and stressful situations that may arise in the course of the legal proceeding.
- To develop agency policies on confidentiality, record keeping, and privileged information.
- To assist other clinicians who may be called to give evidence in a proceeding.

It is our hope that reading this book will increase your comfort with legal processes and legal terminology, also helping you to ask informed questions when seeking legal advice. The practical tips can help you present more effective information as a witness. Since this is not a cookbook, the suggestions should not be followed by rote. When reflecting on how to use our suggestions, consider the assumptions underlying the suggestions and whether these assumptions hold true in your particular situation.

The law and our involvement in legal processes are dynamic. The rules and case law governing testimony of witnesses change over time and across jurisdictions. Yet, while the law is dynamic, any book that addresses how to approach a dynamic system is static. We cannot anticipate how statutes, case law, or codes of ethics will change. We can only discuss what exists today. Many details have been omitted so as not to overwhelm, but also so as not to misinform. Since laws vary both among jurisdictions and over time, we have tried to focus on universal principles. As a witness, you do not need to be an attorney with a 3-year law degree. You may need to hire an attorney to help you understand complicated and changing laws, as well as the specifics of a particular case. Rather than taking the information from this book as absolute, use it to ask questions. For example, you can take the recommendations for preparing reports to your attorney and ask whether she believes these suggestions apply to your situation.

In our attempt to provide interesting, realistic, and thought-provoking examples, some questions and illustrations ask you to ponder choices that verge on the unethical or are, in fact, unethical. Although we ask you to contemplate these types of choices, we ultimately suggest that you act honestly, ethically, and in accordance with the law.

We have tried to make this book readable for nonattorneys. Still, we have occasionally used some legal jargon, which is intended to help you become more conversant with communication in legal arenas. The Glossary at the end of this volume provides definitions of these legal terms, and the Index can be used to find further uses of the terms.

Reading this volume is only one part of preparing to be a witness. You need to become familiar with the current laws governing your area of practice and the legal issues raised in particular cases in which you may be involved. This preparation may entail additional reading, viewing videotapes, participating in training programs, or consulting with a legal expert. Useful sources of information include legal information services, community legal clinics, law schools, and continuing education programs offered by universities, professional associations, professional liability insurance providers, forensic mental health societies, law societies, law libraries at court houses and universities, and associations that govern or promote your profession.

Each attorney may have her own suggestions and advice. If her advice seems inconsistent with something that you have understood from this book, ask questions to try to understand her reasoning. You will be in a better position to heed her advice if you are informed. Your attorney may have her own suggestions for further reading. For example, some attorneys provide witnesses with a memorandum containing suggestions on how to prepare. In the Appendices of this volume, we provide precedents and examples of various documents that you may request or that may be requested of you. Your attorney may be able to comment on these or provide you with additional samples that meet the specific needs of your case and jurisdiction (e.g., reports, affidavits, or transcripts of interviews).

Regardless of the resources you bring to bear, participating effectively in legal processes requires significant informational and emotional preparation. Serving as a witness does not have to be a harrowing experience. We hope this volume will provide you with useful strategies for making the process at least manageable, and possibly even rewarding.

Acknowledgments

Although much of the information in this volume is based upon our experience and readings, we are indebted to many people who have been influential in teaching us about the profoundly interesting interface between law and clinical practice in social work, psychology, and related mental health professions.

Allan thanks the following clinicians and lawyers for sharing their expertise on being a clinician-witness: Deena Mandell, PhD, Marvin Bernstein, LLB, Robin Vogl, MSW, Barbara Landau, LLB, PhD, Barbara Chisholm, MSW, Steve Eichler, LLB, Lisa Estrin, MSW, Julio Arboleda-Florez, MD, and Heather Coleman, PhD. At a personal level, Allan thanks his partner, Greg, for his ongoing support and helpful feedback.

Jon thanks the many people who have contributed to his growth and understanding, and particularly H. D. Kirkpatrick, PhD, Randy Wall, PhD, Rick Deitchman, PhD, Mark Tobin, PhD, Pleas Geyer, MD, Lyn Greenberg, PhD, Jay Flens, PsyD, David Martindale, PhD, Michael Gottlieb, PhD, David Hamilton, Esq., Elizabeth Meadows, MSW, Phyllis Marsh, MA, Billie Maitland, PhD, Chief Judge William G. Jones, Judge Lisa C. Bell, Katie Holliday, Esq., Marsh Jarrell, Sheila Passanant, Esq., William Austin, PhD, Michelle Morris, Esq., and Phil Stahl, PhD. Special thanks go to Jon's family, and particularly to Debra for her understanding and acceptance of the project as well as her husband.

This book is derived from a Canadian version titled *Counsellors as Witnesses*, published by Canada Law Book in 1997. We both thank Howard Davidson and Canada Law Book for their support and feedback on the original version, as well as their generous agreement to grant a license for publication of this U.S.-oriented edition.

Together, Allan and Jon thank Jim Nageotte at The Guilford Press for seeing value in reframing the original book for a U.S. audience. Finally, we extend our appreciation to the copy editor, K. K. Waering, Jr., and the production editor, Anna Nelson at Guilford for their high professional standards and support.

Contents

Prologue

In a precursor to the modern court system, trial by ordeal was used to facilitate justice (Bossy, 1985). For example, trial by hot water required that an accused claiming innocence place one hand in boiling hot water; if, after 3 days, the hand remained unscathed, the accused was declared innocent. Similarly, there were trials by fire, by poison, and by being submerged in cold water to see whether "divine intervention" would intercede, thereby indicating the accused's innocence. Unfortunately, even today's comparatively "civilized" trials are still an ordeal for all too many witnesses. Consider the following examples (each of which references the most relevant chapter in this volume for finding related information):

> Melanie has just graduated with a master's degree in psychology and is ready to take on the world. In one of her first cases she is called upon to testify at a public hearing. The attorney who asks her to testify tells her that she does not have to prepare. She is told that all she has to do is show up and answer the questions as honestly as possible. During the actual testimony, however, Melanie realizes that the attorney is trying to place blame on her for her client's predicament. She feels set up and badgered by the attorney. The judge chastises her for going off on tangents and not answering the questions directly. She wonders, "Did I miss the class when they told us about going to court?" (Chapter 3)

> Erica is a newly hired probation officer. Recently she was responsible for writing a presentence report for a man convicted of gross

1

sexual indecency. Her report included graphic details of his alleged activities. Given her lack of training, she thought the report was only for the judge and attorneys, not realizing that it would become public when entered into the court records. When embarrassing details were released through the media, the man became despondent and attempted suicide. Erica felt responsible for his despair. (Chapter 8)

Joel is a social worker who works with autistic children. The parents of one of Joel's clients felt that the child was not getting any better, and was probably regressing. The parents filed a complaint against Joel with the state social work licensing board. (Chapter 9)

Rebecca is a psychiatrist who reviews the status of patients who have been committed involuntarily to a mental health institution. In preparation for one case, Rebecca was too busy to see the patient personally and relied on reports from the psychologists who had been working with the patient on an ongoing basis. Although the psychologists had recommended that the patient remain in the institution, Rebecca had no firsthand knowledge of the reasons for this recommendation. The court ordered that the patient be released, given the lack of firsthand evidence to indicate whether the client posed a threat to herself or others. (Chapter 7)

Harrison counsels youth who abuse cocaine and other illicit drugs. He keeps excellent clinical records. He also assures his clients that the records are confidential. He is horrified one day when his treatment records are subpoenaed because one of his clients is accused of trafficking. (Chapter 6)

Anders is a counselor who works with refugees. One of his clients was turned down in her initial application for refugee status, and Anders was called to provide information at the appeal. As he was speaking, everyone started to look at him as if they did not understand what he was talking about. Anders suddenly realized he had started to mix up facts from his own family—also immigrants—with facts from his client's family. (Chapter 2)

Danielle was a parent–youth mediator who worked with a court-affiliated diversion program. In her personal life, she was going through separation from a man who mistreated her during their marriage. One day, when she was waiting to be called into court for a child visitation hearing, her estranged husband approached her with a gun. (Chapter 4)

Edna provides therapy for people with AIDS. One of her clients was involved in civil rights litigation, having been fired from his job because of his condition. In preparing her records for the hearing, Edna whited out certain sections of her notes and rewrote them. She submitted a photocopy of the notes so that the whited-out sections could not be seen. One of the attorneys asked for the original copy of her notes, whereupon Edna started to ramble incessantly. The judge asked the attorney, "Can't you control your witness?" (Chapters 4, 5, and 6)

Each of these scenarios is based on a true story. In doing research for this volume, we asked clinicians, "What was your worst experience in relation to a court or similar legal proceeding?" Virtually everyone had at least one memorable story. Some memories were of embarrassing experiences. Some were experiences that revealed a lack of understanding of the legal system. Still others were experiences that pointed to the tension between clinicians safeguarding their client's confidential material and attorneys trying to determine the facts of a case. As a result, these experiences lead some clinicians to avoid courts and attorneys at all cost. Others said that they have learned from their experiences and now feel more comfortable when they are involved in "legal situations." All our colleagues who shared their war stories concurred that they would have preferred not to have learned their lessons solely through trial and error.

This book is our attempt to provide a better understanding of the potential challenges posed to you when interacting with the legal system. There are war stories. There are suggestions. There are warnings. Above all else, we provide a framework of practical information and suggestions for thinking about the tensions between the legal system and clinical practice in psychology, social work, and related professions. This is neither a final nor a definitive work. It will guide and challenge you. It will teach to you think about the tensions between these two dynamic fields of endeavor and ask you to consider who you are and what values you hold dear while also conforming with the legal demands posed by your participating in legal processes.

Chapter 1

Introduction

Clinicians may be called as witnesses in a range of circumstances, from court hearings to private arbitrations to government tribunals (i.e., boards or panels that have quasi-judicial functions). While attorneys have access to a wealth of books and training on how to gather evidence and prepare and examine witnesses, far fewer resources exist for mental health or human service professionals who are called as witnesses. Clinicians are frequently drawn into judicial and quasi-judicial processes with little information about the legal system or their roles as potential witnesses (Gould & Greenberg, 2000; Greenberg, Gould, Gould-Saltman, & Stahl, 2001; Greenberg & Gould, 2001; Madden, 1998). This predicament can be scary and risky. Clinicians' interests may be very different from those of the attorneys who contact them. This book is intended to provide you, the treating therapist or clinician, with an understanding of the legal system, the different roles you might be asked to play as a potential witness, and how to prepare for these varied roles, including how to prepare written reports and other records.

We begin with three simple questions. Who is a clinician? What is a witness? When and why might you be called as a witness?

1. *Who is a clinician?* Clinicians come from varied backgrounds, including social work, psychology, psychiatry, education, criminology, child welfare, nursing, and the clergy (Dickson, 1995). Broadly defined, clinicians provide psychotherapy, personal advice, information, emotional and social support, or problem-solving assistance to their clients. Some disciplines have strict requirements for licensing one to practice.

However, many people who perform clinical services have no formal training and are not regulated under the auspices of a professional organization or a state licensing board. This book deals with issues related to the full spectrum of clinicians. Much of the discussion is applicable across this entire range. Legal and professional role issues that relate to one's training, education, and professional status will be highlighted.

2. *What is a witness?* In common parlance a witness is someone who has observed an event. Within the legal sphere a witness is someone who can provide proof of or attest to a fact or event. Sometimes (as we describe in Chapter 7 on the use of experts), witnesses are asked to provide opinions rather than just facts. Witnesses present information in court and other adjudicative proceedings (i.e., processes in which information is presented to an individual or tribunal that has certain decision-making authority). Many examples in this book use the court as the chief prototype of the adjudicative process. The reason for focusing on court processes is that the court trial is one of the most *formal* types of hearing processes. While full court trials are not the most common type of hearing, other hearings tend to be based on the procedural principles of a trial. If a clinician is prepared for the rigors of a court hearing, she will generally be equipped for less formal processes as well. However, we will also discuss other types of adjudicative processes and identify the different concerns for clinicians involved in these processes. Adjudicative processes can involve multiple parties with overlapping and conflicting interests. To simplify matters, examples used in this book focus on disputes between two parties with adversarial interests.

3. *When and why might you be called as a witness?* Different types of clinicians are more or less likely to find themselves in the position of being called upon as a witness. At one extreme, forensic evaluators are professionals who gather information using a specialized forensic methodology (Austin, 2000, 2001; Gould, 1998, 1999a; Gould & Stahl, 2000; Gould & Bell, 2000) for the express purpose of presenting a forensic interpretation of this information to a court or another legal dispute resolution process. Forensic psychiatrists, for example, may work within the criminal justice system to help the police or state prosecution gather evidence to identify the person who committed a crime. Inquests into the cause of death in a suspected suicide case may require the use of psychological autopsies. Sexual abuse cases may engage a forensic psychologist to conduct a forensic psychological assessment, assisting the police, the court, or an attorney representing the alleged

perpetrator. Traditionally, legal processes relied upon psychiatrists as forensic experts for two reasons. The first is that so-called independent medical examinations (Civil Rule 35) cited the need to use a medical professional. The second is that courts believed that psychiatrists possess a dependable level of expertise given the fact that, as medical professionals, they are subject to a high level of education in the sciences, professional training, role status, and professional regulation.

Since the 1960s, clinicians from other disciplines have gained acceptance as forensic specialists in certain fields of knowledge within their expertise. To economize on resources, some systems have divested responsibilities from traditional doctoral-level trained experts and transferred them to practitioners from disciplines with less advanced degrees who garner lower fees.

Clinicians who work in forensic settings (including psychiatric wards, child protection agencies, and probation and parole offices) can also expect to be called as witnesses as part of their work (Brown & Cox, 1998). These forensic clinicians often have a dual role, raising ethical challenges that are still being debated in the literature (Loewenberg, Dolgoff, & Harrington, 2000; Gould & Greenberg, 2000; Greenberg et al., 2001; Greenberg & Gould, 2001). In a psychiatric facility, for example, forensic clinicians play the role of treating therapist, working with involuntarily committed patients to assist them in regaining their competence or mental health. On the other hand, these same clinicians may be asked to testify about the progress of their patients. Their testimony may take the form of clinical testimony detailing the patient's progress during therapy, or it may entail describing the results of a more formal assessment. The ethical challenge lies in balancing the information needs of the court about the patient's progress with the ethical guidelines about maintaining appropriate boundaries between the role of treating clinician and forensic evaluator. Probation officers, parole officers, hospital-based clinicians, juvenile court clinicians, and child protection workers are the most common types of clinicians with this dual role. A child protection worker, for example, has an obligation to ensure that a child is safe from abuse or neglect. Ideally the worker fulfills this mandate by engaging the family on a voluntary basis while taking on the roles of clinician, support worker, and case manager. To protect the child, however, the worker must also conduct investigations, present information to the court, and monitor the enforcement of court orders.

Clinicians who work outside the legal system may be less likely to be called as witnesses but should be aware of the types of circumstances in which they may be called. Clinical practice with different segments of the population incurs different possibilities of being called as a witness. Clinicians who work with the elderly may be called as witnesses about mental competence in the appointment of trustees for the elder person's property. Clinicians who work with perpetrators or victims of crime may be called in criminal proceedings. Mediators or arbitrators with separating couples may be called as witnesses in child custody and visitation disputes. Clinicians who work with clients with psychiatric disorders may be called for involuntary hospitalization cases. Vocational rehabilitation counselors may be called to provide information in workers' compensation cases. Youth care workers who deal with aggressive clients in residential settings may be subjected to assaults and be called to testify as a victim. The list of examples could go on and on. Unfortunately, some clinicians are afraid to work with psychiatric patients or others where a significant risk of legal involvement may be required. Ethically, clinicians should not discriminate against these groups. Equipped with sufficient legal knowledge and professional competence, clinicians often find that they need not fear this type of work.

In addition to participating in court proceedings, clinicians may be called as witnesses in various forums. Examples of administrative courts and quasi-judicial hearings include social assistance appeals, human rights and discrimination boards, immigration proceedings, public housing appeals, special commissions of inquiry, legislative committees, and criminal injuries compensation boards. Powers vary among administrative court and quasi-judicial forums according to statutes enacted by state legislatures. These powers also vary from state to state. Some tribunals have the power to make only recommendations, while others have the power to make enforceable rulings.

A clinician can become involved in a legal proceeding as a party to an action, as a witness for the court, or as a witness for an attorney. What defines "a party" to a legal proceeding? A party is either the complainant or the recipient of the complaint. A party has a direct stake in the outcome of the case. For example, a client could sue a clinician for malpractice or accuse her of unethical behavior. To defend herself and on the advise of counsel, the clinician may have to be a witness in court or before a professional disciplinary board.

There is an old saying that an attorney who defends himself has a fool as a client. An analogue exists for clinicians. When clinicians attempt to defend themselves before a licensing board or in any legal arena, they operate outside of their professional area of competence. The result may be a less-than-competent defense. Further, there is always concern that when clinicians engage in behavior normally associated with attorneys, the clinician needs to be very careful not to overstep his professional boundaries and engage in functions restricted to those authorized to practice law.

Besides having to defend yourself against charges lodged against you in your role as a clinician, there may be times when you are in the role of plaintiff instead. In other words, you may file a suit against another party. For example, a clinician may find occasion to sue a client to recover unpaid fees for services. Clinicians who work in residential facilities with children may be involved in cases relating to the concept of *in loco parentis* (i.e., acting in the place of a parent). In some situations a party may elect not to be a witness in her own case. However, clinicians need to be aware of potential situations where they may be both a party and a witness. Knowing the ethical issues involved in such dual roles is important. It is often useful to talk with colleagues and request their advice. Communicating immediately with your state licensing board, ethics committee chairperson, and other persons knowledgeable about the ethics of clinical practice is also recommended. Further you could talk with your attorney to shed light on the statutory and/or liability issues involved in engaging in dual roles.

Clinicians who have taken on the role of advocate for a client or social cause may also wish to present themselves as witnesses. Advocates, however, may not make effective witnesses, for reasons we shall discuss. Clinicians need to be aware of the potential conflicts between these roles and the possible ethical dilemmas posed by such advocacy.

Being called as a witness may be unrelated to your work as a clinician. For example, you may witness a crime on the street as a passerby or be personally involved in a landlord–tenant dispute. Although information in this volume may be helpful in preparing you as a witness, in such circumstances you are really a lay witness rather than a witness in your professional capacity. You may actually be a more effective witness if you deemphasize your professional training when you testify in these circumstances.

Ideally, preparation for being a witness in your professional capacity begins before you even begin to offer services. If you have given the matter no thought and instead wait until an incident occurs and then an attorney calls, you will be at a real disadvantage.

To begin preparing for the prospect of being a witness, you need to consider a broad range of issues (see Box).

Role Reflection Questions

- What laws, if any, regulate my profession?
- What professional codes of ethics or standards of professional conduct do I need to follow?
- What are the professional practice guidelines to which I aspire?
- What is the legal mandate, if any, of my agency and my position within that agency? What contractual obligations does my agency have with the government or other funding sources? What agency policies need to be considered?
- Who is my client?
- How does my client view my role? What expectations have I raised about the services I offer, including confidentiality and professional competence?
- What types of conflicts may arise between *my clients and myself*? How likely are these conflicts to escalate beyond informal dispute resolution processes? What can be done to reduce this risk?
- What types of conflicts may arise between *my clients and significant people in their lives*? How likely are these conflicts to escalate beyond informal dispute resolution processes? How likely am I to be brought into these proceedings? What can be done to reduce this risk?
- What is my role as a clinician? What is my role as a witness? What are the potential conflicts between these roles?
- What are my strengths as a potential witness? What do I need to work on?

As you read through this volume, highlight the sections that are relevant to the situations you are most likely to face and identify areas where you need more information. If you work in an agency, undertake with your coworkers and supervisors to develop policies to establish standards of practice. If you are in private practice, consult with colleagues from your profession, as well as legal advisors, to establish rules that govern standards of practice within your private practice. By taking these steps, you will be better equipped to be an effective witness or perhaps even to avoid situations where you will be called as a witness.

Being a witness is not a situation that you should fear or avoid at all costs. A formal hearing may be a constructive or necessary way to deal with certain types of conflict. You may not be able to avoid being called as a witness one day. You may even find that you enjoy this type of work and want to specialize in the area. At least, you can learn how to best tolerate and fulfill your obligations as a witness in a professional manner.

CASE STUDY

The following scenario is used to illustrate issues and strategies *throughout this volume.* For ease of reference, the first initial of each person's name corresponds with the first letter of that person's role in the scenario (P, parent; D, daughter; F, family therapist; M, mediator; L, lawyer; S, social worker; E, evaluator).

Paula Carvey (27 years old) and Philip Carvey (25 years old) have been married for 6 years and are the parents of a 4-year-old daughter, Debra. Although the first 2 years of marriage fulfilled their dreams of wedded bliss, the honeymoon ended when Debra was born. Paula wanted a child at that time, but Philip wanted to wait at least 3 more years. They decided to see a family therapist, Freida, to help them with problems related to trust and communication. Freida used an unorthodox therapy that eventually proved to be ineffective. Paula began to suspect that Philip was having an affair and asked him to leave the home. Philip left, but immediately sought the services of an attorney, Lori, to help him win custody of Debra and to move back into the family home. Lori referred Philip and Paula to a mediator, Michael, to help them work out their differences on an amicable basis. During mediation, Paula accused Philip of sexually abusing Debra. Michael said that he could not continue mediation with outstanding allegations of abuse, so he encouraged Paula to call child protection services if she were truly concerned about Debra's safety. Paula called and Sam was assigned as a social work investigator for the case. Sam conducted an investigation and met with Debra, but could not substantiate abuse. He suggested that the Carveys undergo a custody evaluation, thinking that this would help resolve their

> domestic dispute and hoping that the assessor would pick up any incidents of abuse. Philip and Paula agreed to hire Evelyn to perform the evaluation.

If you have worked on divorce and custody cases, the multiplicity of players involved in this scenario is familiar; for others, the case may seem like a Russian novel, with so many characters to keep track of. Understanding the respective role of each player, and the issues each player may present to you, will enable you to make clearer decisions about how to wind your way through a legal proceeding.

COURT AND OTHER ADJUDICATIVE HEARINGS

In order to provide an overview of adjudicative proceedings, we will give generic descriptions of court and other adjudicative processes. You will need to expand this outline by learning about the specific processes in your jurisdiction and in the types of hearings where you may be called as a witness. Administrators, clerks, attorneys, and experienced clinicians who work within these systems are often the best sources of information.

When people are faced with conflict, they can deal with it in various ways. For example, they may avoid the conflict, accommodate the other person, engage in a physical fight, seek compromise, collaborate, negotiate, argue, or problem-solve (Mayer, 2000). In most situations the decision to go to court or adjudication to resolve the conflict is made when parties have exhausted less formal and legalistic dispute resolution processes. In the case example, Paula and Philip have tried to deal with their marital conflict by several appropriate means. They have sought therapy. After the decision to separate and gain legal counsel, they have attempted a mediated solution. These solutions did not solve the conflict. Suddenly, with no historical foundation to expect an allegation, Paula accuses Philip of sexually abusing their child. Now, the familial conflict escalates significantly. The father is not allowed to visit with his child under a judge's protection order, put into effect until completion of the state's child protection investigation. The mother talks with the child about the alleged events perpetrated by her father. The child begins to change how she views her father, becoming increasingly angry and distrusting of a father who would abuse his child. The attorneys fire off letters to each other, accusing the other side of playing games with the system. The investigation takes about 8 months to complete, and the result is a recommendation for a comprehensive child custody evaluation. The judge orders the evaluation and schedules a hearing for 4 months later. To protect the child, the court directs the father into supervised visitation with the child for 2 hours a week.

Whether you are a clinician or a party to an action, many people who become embroiled in legal battles have little information about the actual workings of legal processes. Portrayals of trials on television and in other media often convey misleading impressions. The court process can take months or even years, rather than 2 hours in a movie or half an hour in a sitcom. Even live telecasts of real cases can be deceptive. You only observe what happens in the courtroom, and only a small percentage of cases—those with "juicy" issues or popular appeal—end up on television. You do not see many of the mundane elements of legal proceedings, the private negotiations, or the real impact of the process on the parties involved. As a clinician preparing to be a witness, watching courtroom dramas provides limited value beyond entertainment. If Lori were representing Philip in divorce proceedings, she would not likely have the opportunity to play to the cameras or to make millions from the book rights.

CONCEPTS OF JUSTICE AND PROCEDURAL FAIRNESS

Conceptually, adjudicative proceedings are designed to be places where people can go to have their disputes dealt with in a just manner. Information is presented to an impartial judge or tribunal. In our public court system the doctrine of *stare decisis* is applied, so that "like cases are treated alike." Judges are guided by precedents. A precedent is a legal principle established in previous decisions made by higher courts such as state or federal appellate or supreme courts. Judges are guided also by laws passed by government. Requiring judges to follow strict legal rules ensures that people are treated equally and are not at the mercy of the unfettered whims or politics of the decision maker (Satterfield & Vayda, 1997). Judicial discretion, however, may be required to ensure that people are treated equitably rather than equally. Judges may be able to rule differently on similar cases by distinguishing the facts of each case. Just because one family counselor using an unorthodox therapy was found liable for malpractice in one case does not mean that Freida must be held liable for malpractice. The situation could be different, and her unorthodox intervention warranted. Legal principles are developed by courts in the process of discovering similarities and differences among cases (Albert, 2000). Even when governments pass legislation and codify the law, judges may still exercise discretion in how they interpret and apply the law to various situations.

Procedural rules are designed to ensure that the process is fair. For example, each party is given notice of the issues to be raised in a case and provided with an opportunity to present its information and argument. Each party can also use legal representation. The decision maker(s) must be neutral or impartial. Courts and other tribunals are based on an adversarial process in which each party has the responsibility for presenting and arguing its side of the case. The underlying premise of an adversarial process is that by having each party present its strongest case and challenge the case it opposes, truth is more likely to emerge. One aspect of procedural regulation is the law of evidence. This law defines what information may be introduced into court, how it may be introduced, and how it may be used in the decision-making process. Although attorneys have the primary responsibility for determining what evidence to call and how to call it, witnesses can be better prepared to provide effective testimony if they are familiar with some of the key laws of evidence.[1] As a forensic evaluator,[2] Evelyn knows that there is a good chance her custody report could be used in court and will ensure that the report meets required legal standards.

In most court hearings a single judge is the sole decision maker. In some cases involving serious allegations, such as murder, the case may be tried by a judge and jury. In these cases the jury is charged with the duty of determining which facts presented by the parties are more likely to be true. The judge is responsible for determining pro-

---

[1]Evidence codes of states are generally based upon both state legislative statutes and the state's adaptation of the Federal Rules of Evidence. All states have evidence codes that determine how the court should define an expert, a fact witness, the limitations of expert testimony, etc.; see Shuman and Sales (1998) and Krauss and Sales (1999).

[2]Sometimes referred to as a "custody assessor." Often differences in language stem from different professional orientations. For instance, social workers use the term "assessment," while as psychologists use "evaluation" or psychiatrists use "diagnosis." Although each term is related, they have different meanings within the professions.

cedural and legal issues. In a trial by judge alone, the judge is responsible for factual, legal, and procedural issues. In child custody proceedings for the Carveys, the legal issues could include how to interpret family laws regarding the best interests of the child. Whether Philip was an abusive parent would be a factual issue. How Paula's testimony about sexual abuse could be brought into court would be a procedural issue.

The admissibility of evidence and the weight given to evidence are dealt with as two separate issues. The question of whether to allow Evelyn to testify about her report, for example, is an admissibility issue. Once the judge admits her as an expert, then she is allowed to provide opinions about the family system. These opinions are drawn from the information gathered during her evaluation. The clearer the reliability, relevance, and helpfulness of the conclusions in Evelyn's report, the more weight (or value) the judge gives to her testimony (Krauss & Sales, 1999). Since family matters are tried by a judge alone, the judge would have responsibility for all of these decisions. In cases tried by a jury, the judge determines admissibility and the jury determines what weight to give to the testimony.

INITIATING THE PROCESS

If you think about the broad range of conflicts that arise in human interaction, relatively few end up in court. Even among cases that are filed in court, less than 10% result in a full trial of the issues. A wide variety of formal and informal processes goes on before a trial takes place. As a potential witness, how you act during the pretrial stages can increase or decrease the chance that the case will go to trial and that you will be called as a witness.

If we take the juncture at which Philip called his attorney as the point where the legal process began, there are still a number of opportunities for the case to be resolved before trial. Although many people conceive of attorneys as predatory hawks who are ever eager to take a case to court, attorneys do have an ethical obligation to try to resolve disputes in the most constructive and cost-effective manner possible. Attorneys may negotiate for settlement on behalf of their clients or call upon the services of other professionals to help resolve the issues. Lori could contact Freida to explore information Freida gathered in family therapy.[3] This information may help Lori to determine the prospects of Philip and Paula reconciling their marriage or to identify facts that would help Lori negotiate a custody arrangement that is favorable to her client, Philip. On the facts provided, Lori contacted Michael to help mediate the case.[4] Because of their involvement with the family, both Freida and Michael could be witnesses if the matter of child custody could not be resolved through negotiation or mediation.

If a client decides to take the case to court, the documents filed in court must identify the relevant parties and a legal cause of action. The cause of action identifies the legal grounds under which a case is brought to court. For example, if the police were to charge Philip with sexual assault on a minor, he would be identified as the defendant and the state would be identified as the prosecutor. If Paula were to sue Freida for malpractice, Paula would be identified as the plaintiff and Freida as the defendant.

Different documents are required to initiate different legal processes, whether it be a claim for a civil law suit, a petition for divorce, and so on.[5] These documents give the defending party notice of the allegations made and remedies sought. The party against whom the charge is made is given an opportunity to submit his own documents stating his defense. This provides the initiating party notice of whether and how the defending party intends to respond to the allegations. As will be described later on, potential witnesses may be asked to submit sworn affidavits in this exchange of documents, in support of the position of one or the other parties. Witnesses are also important at this stage in

---

[3]Some states have statutory limitations on what a marriage clinician may provide to one side in a legal dispute. There also may be ethical issues involved in releasing information about marriage counseling to one side without the express written permission of the other side. Consult an attorney for your state's statutes and your state association for the ethical responsibilities you have in such a context.

[4]Some jurisdictions have mandatory mediation, meaning that parties must try to mediate their dispute before they are allowed to go to trial. Typically both attorneys contact the mediator rather than having initial contact from only one side. This avoids the appearance of the mediator's having been inappropriately influenced by one side prior to the beginning of mediation. Also, there are several ethical issues pertaining to the admissibility of testimony from a mediator. Check with your state association as well as colleagues in your community. There are times when there are clearly defined local rules as well as clearly defined informal jurisdiction-specific rules about certain types of testimony. Knowing these community standards may be very useful. For a discussion of the progress on the draft Uniform Mediation Act, see http://acresolution.org.

[5]Terminology for names of documents varies across states and other jurisdictions.

helping each side know whether it has a good case and whether there is room for settlement outside of court.

PRETRIAL PROCESSES

Once a case is filed in court, parties may engage in a range of pretrial processes conducted by judges or other officers of the court:

Motions

Each side may bring motions to court to deal with procedural or *interim* issues (i.e., issues that require a temporary decision until a final decision can be reached). Motions generally do not involve testimony from nonparty witnesses, but written evidence may be used in support of a motion (e.g., a sworn statement from Evelyn recommending interim custody of Debra).

Disclosures

Although Hollywood productions of courtroom drama are filled with surprise witnesses and testimony, real court cases produce few courtroom surprises, since each party has an obligation to disclose its case to the other side.[6] As a witness, you may be asked to provide written information (including case files) or to submit to an oral examination prior to trial.

Mini-Trials, Preliminary Inquiries, and Pretrial Settlement Conferences

Different jurisdictions and types of cases may offer or require different pretrial proceedings to try to resolve cases amicably or efficiently. Pretrials can speed up the process by helping the parties to identify whether a reasonable cause of action exists or what the likely outcome of a full trial would be. If a trial is unavoidable, pretrial conferences can narrow the issues and streamline how the trial will be conducted. Wit-

---

[6]Some states have no pretrial discovery rules for family court cases.

nesses may be called in mini-trials and preliminary inquiries, but generally only the parties and their attorneys attend settlement conferences.

The parties may also decide to resolve the case through other conflict resolution processes, such as attorney-led negotiation, mediation or arbitration. Clinicians may be asked to participate in mediation or arbitration. Arbitrations can require you to attend, but participation of witnesses is voluntary in most informal dispute resolution processes. Your participation in such processes could affect whether you are called to testify in a subsequent trial. You need to know the parameters of the dispute resolution process that you are being asked to participate in. Information presented in some processes is restricted from use in certain other legal proceedings. For other processes the information is not restricted.

THE TRIAL

After a case is calendared for trial,[7] the procedures still vary for different types of hearings. The following outline is intended to provide an overview. Details may vary in your specific jurisdiction.

First, the attorneys for each party present their opening arguments and identify facts they intend to prove. Following the opening arguments, each party presents various forms of evidence to try to prove its case. The party initiating the action, the plaintiff, is first to present its case. In a child protection proceeding, for example, the attorney for the protection agency could call Sam to testify about information gathered in his investigation of abuse allegations against Philip. The plaintiff's attorney begins her questioning of Sam. This is called an "examination-in-chief" or "direct examination." Philip's attorney then has the opportunity to ask Sam questions in what is called a "cross-examination."[8] The agency attorney has another opportunity to ask Sam questions in

---

[7]Courts use the term "calendared" to refer to scheduling. A trial is normally calendared for a particular trial term. Trial terms typically range from 2–3 weeks. If your trial is calendared for the April 30th trial term and is listed on the calendar as trial number 10, this means that nine other proceedings are scheduled before your trial can begin. Whether the court will hear your case during that particular term depends upon how quickly the cases scheduled before yours are resolved.

[8]There may be more than two attorneys. For instance, the court may appoint a guardian *ad litem* to act as attorney for the child.

the "redirect examination" (as does the defense attorney, in the "recross-examination"). Each type of examination has particular purposes, rules, and strategies.

In addition to oral testimony, you may be asked to provide documentary evidence. For clinicians, the most typical documents requested are evaluations, psychosocial assessments, progress notes, business records, and psychological test results.[9] Another form of evidence is "real evidence" (artifacts, videotapes, audiotapes, photographs, or other objects). For example, photographs of scars or bruising could be used in support of allegations of abuse or assault.

After the party initiating the proceedings presents its case, the responding party has the opportunity to call its evidence. As with the initiating party, the responding party examines the witnesses it calls, and the initiating party has the opportunity to cross-examine them. When both parties have completed presenting their evidence, each party provides its closing arguments. If the trial is by jury, then the judge provides a charge (or instructions) to the jury, summarizing the evidence presented, outlining the factual questions the jury is to answer, and clarifying any legal issues. The jury meets privately to consider the questions and make its findings of fact. If the trial is by judge alone, then the judge makes these findings.

DECIDING

The decisions of a court are based upon both the "burden of proof" and the "standard of proof." Burden of proof refers to which party has the primary responsibility of proving its case, whereas the "standard of proof" refers to the degree of certainty that the party with the burden of proof must provide. The burden and standards of proof differ for different types of cases. In family law and most civil proceedings, the party bringing the ac-

---

[9]The release of psychological test data may involve only the release of *raw* data to another mental health expert competent to interpret the test results. Consult your ethics requirements before releasing any psychological test data. Even when the court orders the release of the data, it is important that you take steps to educate the court about your ethical obligations. Once you have formally made your concerns known to the court, if the court still insists upon release of the test data, you are obliged to release the data. Be sure there is a signed court order directing you to do so. When uncertain, always consult your state board or association as well as a knowledgeable attorney.

tion to court has the responsibility to prove its case "on the preponderance of the evidence." In other words, the initiating party must prove that its version of the facts is more likely to have occurred than not. In criminal proceedings, the prosecution must prove its case "beyond a reasonable doubt." Each criminal offense has particular legal components that must be proven. If the accused can raise a reasonable doubt that one of these elements may not have happened, then she must be found not guilty. She does not need to prove she is innocent (Myers, 1993). As a result, criminal prosecutions require much stronger evidence than civil proceedings. The reason for this high standard of proof is to ensure that a person is not convicted of an offense she did not commit. The downside is that some people who commit offenses will be set free because the prosecution could not meet the high standard of proof.

Once the findings of fact have been reported to the court, the judge decides upon the legal consequences of the findings. If a person has been found guilty of a criminal offense, the judge will receive oral or written submissions, sometimes called "arguments" or "briefs," to help in deciding on the appropriate sentence. If Philip were convicted of sexual assault, then the court may consider a psychological report prepared either by a court-affiliated worker (e.g., a probation officer) or a forensic mental health expert such as a psychologist or psychiatrist. If Freida were found legally responsible for malpractice, then the judge would need to determine the appropriate remedy, such as monetary compensation for damages and/or pain and suffering.

APPEALS

Trial court decisions are sometimes appealed to a higher court. The person bringing the appeal must argue that either an error of law or a procedural error was made at trial. For example, it might be argued that the judge misinterpreted the laws on child custody or permitted irrelevant and prejudicial information to be heard.[10] There may be a "case of first impression" in which a point of law has not been dealt with previously and the judge is asked to establish a new precedent.

---

[10]In order to understand the important differences between "testimony that is probative" and "testimony that is prejudicial" for a particular case, you may need to consult an attorney.

When a case is appealed, it is heard by an appellate court judge or a small panel of judges. During an appeal, the facts of a case are not re-tried. There are no witnesses and no new evidence. The appellate court examines the record of the trial court. The judges may refer to transcripts, evidence presented at trial, and exhibits prepared for and admitted during trial. This is one reason why it is important for clinicians to prepare thorough reports. Although oral testimony may be limited to that which is presented during direct and cross-examination, a comprehensive report may provide the appeals court with valuable information that was not presented during oral testimony at trial. As long as the trial court admitted your report into evidence, the appellate court is allowed to review it. During the appeal, the attorney for each party presents written and/or oral arguments to the court. If the appealing party wins, the appeals court may substitute its own order or refer the case back to the trial court to be retried. If the appeal is lost, then the trial court judgment stands.

OTHER TRIBUNALS

Noncourt tribunals vary in their levels of formality. Their processes are defined by their enabling legislation and regulations. As a prospective witness, your role may be quite different in a human rights hearing than in a professional discipline hearing. Although processes vary, most retain basic rights of procedural fairness: notice of the charges, a right to be heard, and an impartial decision maker. Some tribunals use only written submissions because oral testimony tends to be more time-consuming and costly. Often, the most important function of a clinician as a witness is providing written reports rather than oral testimony.

Use of attorneys may be encouraged or discouraged at different types of hearings. Some processes discourage the use of attorneys to keep the process informal and to minimize costs. Informal proceedings tend to be more accessible to the public. If Paula were concerned about Freida's conduct as a family counselor, she could sue Freida for malpractice in court or bring a complaint to her professional regulatory body. Paula is more likely to complain to the professional body because its process is less formal and less costly.

Whereas courts have a fixed adjudicative function and process, other bodies often have overlapping functions. For example, some human rights commissions develop their own policies, giving them both law-making and adjudicative functions. Legislative committees use hearings primarily for informing their law-making functions. Other bodies have enforcement as well as adjudicative functions. Some bodies, such as an ombuds, can make recommendations but lack direct powers to make and enforce decisions. Some bodies are more investigative than adjudicative.

Investigative models are often used as a method of Alternative Dispute Resolution, where the parties agree to submit their issues to an alternative forum to the public court system. In an investigative model, the decision maker is more active than a judge in collecting information and questioning witnesses. An investigative model is a process that many clinicians who perform psychosocial assessments will be familiar with. For example, in conducting a custody assessment, Evelyn would conduct home visits, interview and observe each family member with each child, and gather information from collateral information sources such as family members, pediatricians, teachers, youth clinicians, neighbors, and others who have direct observational knowledge of the children and their relationship with each parent (Austin, 2001; Gould, 1998, Gould & Bell, 2000). In contrast to a judge, an investigative decision maker is bound by the scope of her investigative powers rather than rules concerning what evidence can be heard. Your role as a witness in an investigative proceeding is vastly different from that in an adjudicative or legislative hearing.

Different tribunals have different focal points of inquiry. Criminal proceedings, compensation cases, and disciplinary proceedings tend to focus on the past. As a fact witness, you may be asked about your knowledge of what happened and who did what. As an expert witness, you may be asked to hypothesize about the likelihood of certain events and their effects on another event, either an expert opinion about a past event or a prediction about a future one (Austin, 2001). As an expert witness, you also may be asked to opine about what kind of punishment or restitution is required to compensate for any wrongful acts committed. In custody, access, child protection, and legislative proceedings, the focus is on the future. Although the past may be used to inform decisions about the future, you may be asked for opinions about what needs to be done in the future for the best interests of the child, the community, and so on. Such predictions should be based upon the science of

your discipline, such as the research in the behavioral science literature.[11] Certain forums such as legislative hearings allow for the presentation of one's political beliefs and values as well as science, while other
types of hearings may limit your involvement to the presentation of
"facts."

OVERVIEW

This chapter raises far more questions and challenges than it presents
answers. The rest of this volume provides information and strategies on:

- How to respond when you are first contacted by an attorney.
- What to discuss when meeting with an attorney.
- How to maintain records.
- How to prepare reports and affidavits.
- How to prepare for oral testimony.
- How to present oral testimony.
- The role of an expert witness.
- How to deal with malpractice and professional complaints.

Undoubtedly more questions will be raised. The proceedings will now
come to order.

---

[11]Providing the court with opinions based on behavioral science literature is the proper role of
an expert witness. As Shuman and Sales (1998) suggest, the court is but poorly served when
expert witnesses offer personal opinion and clinical judgment in the guise of science. A similar
argument is offered by Lavin and Sales (1998) when they debate the moral foundation of expert witness testimony.

Chapter 2

Beginning with Yourself

For many clinicians, the legal process is foreign, frightening, or despised. Clinicians may feel patronized and disempowered by attorneys. Part of a clinician's aversion to participating in the legal arena may be due to a lack of familiarity with the legal process. Other aspects are related to real differences between the professional philosophies and perspectives embodied in the training and experiences of clinicians and attorneys. To be effective as a witness, you need to identify any sources of frustration that you may have with legal processes. Awareness of these issues can help you with the same type of "conscious use of self" as a witness as your awareness of self would serve you in therapeutic interactions with your clients (Schetky & Colbach, 1982).

Effective clinicians conduct their work by making deliberate and informed choices about how to present themselves, what to say, and how to say it. This notion of the intentional professional applies whether the clinician is diagnosing a client, performing therapy, or acting as a witness (Schon, 1990). Just as you must "begin with yourself" when working in a clinical practice role (Hunt, 1976), you must also begin with yourself when your profession takes you into the role of a witness. This reflective process starts with your asking yourself:

- What are my *experiences* with the legal system?
- What *attitudes and triggers* have I developed because of these experiences?
- What are my professional *roles*?
- What *commonalties and conflicts* exist between attorneys and myself?

With this awareness and understanding, you will be better able to act and react intentionally to situations where you are in contact with the legal system.

EXPERIENCES, ATTITUDES, AND TRIGGERS

Our values and attitudes toward attorneys and the legal system are shaped by both positive and negative experiences. Such experiences can take a number of forms. A key experience could be a childhood recollection, a relationship with someone who works within the legal system, or prior interaction with the legal system in your role as a clinician. From childhood, do you remember images of attorneys as virtuous champions of justice or as self-righteous hawks and victimizers? How have movies and other media shaped your views of the legal system? What horror stories have you heard? What roles have important people in your life played in relation to the legal system, whether judges, attorneys, victims, experts, offenders, policemen, or mediators? Have you ever been called to court or to a professional disciplinary hearing to testify? How did you feel you were treated?

Many clinicians are troubled by their entry into the legal system. Attorneys are trained in the art of adversarial exchange. They appear prepared to spend days or weeks on end in the courtroom, battling with their colleagues over legal issues. They challenge. They argue. They play strategic games with the facts. In the courtroom, attorneys zealously advocate for their client's position and work hard at undermining the credibility of the other side. When the trial is over, most attorneys shake hands and leave the adversarial spirit in the courtroom.

Clinicians seem to have thinner skin. Most of us are not trained in the art of advocacy, nor do we spend our professional time in an adversarial setting. We expect empathy, honesty, concern, and support from our colleagues. Our training compels us to be gentle, compassionate, understanding, forgiving, and constructive in our communications. Such professional expectations about communication and collegial treatment may serve us poorly when we enter the legal arena.

In psychological terms, "countertransference" refers to an unconscious process where work with a client triggers feelings in the clinician related to important people or relationships in the clinician's personal life. If the clinician is aware of her countertransference, she will be in a better position to ensure that it does not hinder her effectiveness as a witness (Schetky & Colbach, 1982; Goldstein, 1988). Consider feelings evoked by the legal process that may stem from prior experiences. For example, if Michael has had horrible experiences with authority in the past, he may feel scared, anxious, or angry when dealing with an authoritative attorney or tribunal. Unchecked, these feelings may cause Michael to become unduly passive or, alternatively, argumentative with an attorney. Countertransference could also occur in relation to the substantive issues of a legal dispute. For example, Sam could have unresolved issues regarding aggression or sexual abuse from his own background. If Sam becomes involved in child protection proceedings with the Carveys, he needs to ensure that his personal feelings do not bias his ability to provide a proper assessment.

Personal reflection is just one way to deal with countertransference as a witness. Maintaining a personal log or self-check questionnaire may help to raise your awareness of how a particular case or dealing with particular legal professionals is affecting you: What feelings does this case evoke in me; where are these feelings coming from; to what extent are they related to the actual case versus events in my own life; how do they affect my behavior in the courtroom? In situations where countertransference may have a significant impact on your ability to present as a witness, further exploration with a peer, supervisor, or therapist may be required.

Countertransference can also positively affect a clinician's performance as a witness. Some clinicians enjoy the attention of being asked for their advice. They may have had aspirations of becoming an attorney at one point in their lives and thrive on the opportunity to participate in legal processes. Other clinicians, consciously or unconsciously, use their emotion-tinged responses to convey genuine passion and conviction in giving their testimony.

ROLES

In a prototypical adjudicative process, the primary issue to be decided is whose version or interpretation of the facts is to be believed as the truth. From this determination, the adjudicator can decide on the appropriate disposition or remedy. An effective witness in this adjudicative process is someone who can communicate facts and opinions about those facts in a credible manner. A credible witness is one in whom the adjudicator is more likely to believe. Qualities that tend to convey credibility include candor, openness, honesty, frankness, impartiality, trustworthiness, respectfulness, knowledge, and confidence. To be an effective witness, one must not only possess these qualities but also be *perceived* to possess these qualities. Credibility as a witness is akin to one of the core conditions of clinical practice, that is, genuineness (Ivey & Ivey, 1999). Professional clinicians know that to be effective as a clinician they need to convey authenticity to their clients—otherwise, the clinician cannot develop a positive working alliance with the client. Similarly, a clinician cannot be effective as a witness unless she develops a relationship based on credibility with the decision maker(s) in the adjudicative process.

Lay witnesses are generally provided with no more than two pages of tips on how to be an effective witness. So why does a clinician need a whole book? In one sense, clinicians are already at an advantage, since honesty is a professional ethic, and clinicians are practiced in the conscious use of self. *Being credible* does not seem that hard. In the legal system, *being credible* is not enough. You must be *perceived* as credible. That is where the adversarial nature of the legal system sometimes confounds well-meaning clinicians.

The legal system presents many challenges to clinicians. On the one hand, during direct examination, there is an interest in obtaining a description of the facts as you know them. After you complete your direct examination, however, there is an opportunity for the other side to ask questions, too. This cross-examination is aimed at undermining your testimony from direct examination or making that testimony less credible. Further complicating matters are the multiple roles that clinicians play and the variety of proceedings with which clinicians may be involved. While the temptation to seek out a simple cookbook-style recipe for being an effective witness is great, your experience in legal proceedings can be much more influential and fulfilling if you take sufficient time and care to become an informed and intentional participant.

A vital first step in becoming an intentional witness is to identify your roles. Some roles may be *required*. Others may be of your choosing, based on professional and personal preferences. Consider Freida and Sam. Freida is a family therapist who works in a private practice setting with people who voluntarily attend. Freida has no ongoing relationship with legal systems. Sam is a social worker who works in a forensic setting and is directly involved with the child protection system. Although their roles as clinicians and witnesses have some similarities, significant differences also exist.

As clinicians, both Freida and Sam are likely to view themselves as helping professionals, agents of change, and advocates for their clients. While Freida operates in private practice and determines her own role, Sam works in the context of an agency mandated to safeguard children from abuse and neglect. Accordingly, Sam must be aware of his dual role and of conflicts that arise when voluntary interventions are insufficient to ensure the welfare of a child. Given these contexts, Sam and Freida have significantly different orientations toward the legal system. Their orientation will affect the way they keep records, their relationship with attorneys, and the way they present evidence.

As a custody evaluator, Evelyn has been appointed by the court to gather information from multiple data sources, form her opinions, and present a report. She should neither provide therapy to nor mediate with Philip and Paula, since this could compromise her role as an evaluator (Gould, 1998; Greenberg & Shuman, 1997). However, the manner in which Evelyn conducts her assessment may have therapeutic or mediative effects. For instance, the manner in which she drafts her assessment could include conciliatory language and highlight the strengths of each parent. The lines between therapy, mediation, and assessment are not always clear (Greenberg & Shuman, 1997; Gould & Greenberg, 2000; Greenberg et al., 2001). Still, a reflective practitioner needs to be aware of the boundaries that her role entails as well as to have an understanding of the role limitations that can affect the scope of her testimony.

COMMONALITIES, CONFLICTS, AND MOVING BEYOND

Although clinicians and attorneys often feel at odds with one another, they have a substantial set of values and methods in common. Attorneys and clinicians have common interests in client rights, advocacy, and justice (Lynch & Mitchell, 1995). Although their definitions and modes of implementation may be different, their ethical commitments are similar. For example, both disciplines seek to educate others about political and human issues. Both endeavor to influence people with power to protect the interests of minorities, victims, and the disadvantaged (National Association of Social Workers, 2001).

Evelyn might find it personally gratifying that her assessments influence important decisions about Debra's welfare. Acting as a witness in one proceeding not only affects the welfare of an individual client but also can have much broader policy implications and affect the lives of many other people (Lukton, 1978). If Evelyn were to provide convincing information about research pertaining to identification of sexual abuse in young children, this research could establish a precedent that would affect how child protection authorities dealt with future cases. Clinicians may take pleasure from work in legal processes because of personal interests. Freida may enjoy public speaking. Sam may enjoy working with Lori because of his admiration for attorneys such as fictional television character, Ally McBeal. Evelyn may take satisfaction from responding well in a cross-examination, demonstrating that her assessment was well founded. Clinicians may even find that their experience in legal proceedings provides them with new insights to take back to their clinical work (Barker & Branson, 1993).

A clinician must use a different set of skills and orientation to function effectively in adjudicative processes. However, some of the traditional attributes of clinicians will be helpful in pursuing alternatives to adjudicative processes. If Michael uses his mediation skills effectively, he can help the parties resolve custody and access on a consensual, amicable basis. If Evelyn produces a sound evaluation, Lori can use this evaluation to negotiate terms of a separation agreement. A clinician's communication skills will be beneficial in all types of legal proceedings.

Unfortunately, not all clinical approaches are easily transferable to legal processes. Involvement in them is not necessarily easy or gratifying. You may feel anxious because your work is being put on trial. You may feel ridiculed or demeaned by how attorneys question you. You may become frustrated with the legal process because of a lack of control over it. If you see your role as case management or facilitation, legal proceedings can usurp that role. You may find it frustrating to operate as a mere "functionary" for the legal system (Lynch & Mitchell, 1995). As a witness, you may find that you cannot act as an advocate or helping agent for your client. Because attorneys tend to control the process, you may feel that your role is diminished to that of a passive collaborator. You may not have time for the legal requirements of documentation for day-to-day record keeping and court proceedings. Delays within the justice system and the stress of legal proceedings will affect both you and your client. You may not be properly compensated for your time. The language used by attorneys may sound obscure or convoluted. Your participation in a controversial legal dispute can bring negative responses from colleagues or clients. You may even be followed down the street by a journalist who is researching a current case, only to be vilified on the 6 o'clock news. Some of these issues can be dealt with once you understand them. Others have no easy solution.

The relationship between a clinician and attorney is often either a love or hate relationship, depending on each person's personal as well as professional experiences with one another. Certainly, the legal profession is made up of both ethical and unethical, competent, and incompetent practitioners; likewise for mental health and related professions. As a potential witness, you may have the opportunity to forge successful working relationships with like-minded attorneys, but you will need to learn how to work with the full gamut of possible attorneys to effectively fulfill your roles as clinician and witness.

The following discussion outlines six conflicts between legal and clinical approaches, offering suggestions for how a clinician can deal with these conflicts

Adversarial versus Collaborative Approaches

Clinicians work collaboratively with client systems to resolve problems in ways that foster client self-determination. While attorneys work collaboratively with their own clients, adjudication uses an adversarial process that pits one attorney's client against another's. Adjudication generally results in win–lose outcomes. Decision-making authority is placed in the hands of a judge or third-party decision maker rather than the client and/or the clinician. Incarceration for criminal activities and involuntary committals to mental health institutions exemplify the extent to which legal systems can interfere with self-determination. Whereas attorneys have traditionally had a rights orientation, clinicians tend to be more relationship-oriented.

When you testify against a client in a legal proceeding, your working relationship can be hurt or even severed entirely. However, providing evidence may not be, in and of itself, the problem. A number of other factors contribute to the impact of testifying. Have you clearly identified your role to your client and the possibility that you could be called to testify? Is the agreement about your role in writing and signed by you and your client? Have you properly identified the limits of confidentiality? Are the limits of confidentiality clearly described in a written document signed by you and your client? Have you and the client already tried to resolve matters through less formal and adversarial means? Did you make real-time accurate notes about these discussions and the options proposed to avoid the litigation?

If you do have to present evidence at a hearing, the manner in which you do so is all-important (see Chapter 5). When caught up in the adversarial spirit of a proceeding, a clinician may end up presenting information in a divisive, provocative, or aggravating manner. Even though the legal process has adversarial components, a clinician is normally most effective as a witness when providing balanced, matter-of-fact information. Evelyn's written assessment will be more influential in a legal proceeding if she focuses on objective facts. "I observed that when Paula said she would not allow Philip to have access to Debra, Philip said he would abduct Debra" would be a more influential statement than "Philip cannot be trusted because he plans to abduct Debra." Through direct and concrete statements, the clinician will seem more credible not only to the decision maker, but also to the client, both of whom may sense greater truth in the information that you have provided.

In some situations, clinicians make use of the authoritative nature of legal processes in order to facilitate therapeutic change (Palmer, 1983). For example, child protection workers such as Sam can use the authority of the court as part of a planned intervention to ensure that a child is protected from an abusive parent. Although clinicians prefer to work with clients on a voluntary and consensual basis, limits on self-determination exist when there is a risk of harm to the client or others. Some clinicians who work with involuntary clients feel that they, the clinicians, have too much authority; while other clinicians feel they have too little authority.

As a clinician, you can temper your authority and strive to work with a client on a more consensual basis by trying to work out a voluntary plan of action prior to going to court. If you cannot come to an agreement with the client, you can try to help him understand his emotional reactions to the legal consequences of his actions so that he can make an informed choice about how to respond. You can also help your client think through different options and how those options might have very different emotional consequences for him.

You cannot and should not interpret legal decisions for your client or provide legal advice. However, it is appropriate to assist your client in developing a better understanding of her feelings about different legal options. You may also be helpful in guiding your client to ask questions of her attorney which would serve to better clarify her understanding of the legal consequences of her choices and decisions.

If you are going to be a witness in a case involving your clients, you need to explain your role to them as early as possible.[1] To the extent that you are honest with them up front, they will be able to make their own choices about whether and how to cooperate with you. Further, they will not be surprised if you do raise evidence against them.

Clinicians representing disadvantaged groups may find the legal system oppressive. They may be concerned about the negative impact of an adversarial process on their clients or find that the law contains systemic biases. For example, some domestic violence clinicians who work with abused women find that criminal procedure favors the rights of the accused over the rights of their clients. Accordingly, such clinicians may be reluctant to cooperate with the legal system. Conversely, some clinicians who work with men accused of perpetrating violence might be reluctant to support the legal system because they may believe there is a bias favoring the rights of victims over the rights of alleged perpetrators.

Certainly, problems do exist. Clinicians can play a significant role in challenging injustices and advocating for change within the limits of their professional roles. However, before a clinician decides not to cooperate as a witness, she needs to be aware of the potential consequences of taking certain actions. In the extreme, refusing to cooperate can result in charges of obstructing justice or contempt of court (see Chapter 3). If faced with this issue, you need to weigh the risks and benefits of refusing to participate in the process with the risks and benefits of cooperating. Consult your profession's ethical standards and codes of conduct and seek the advice of colleagues. You may need to consult with not only your personal attorney but with an attorney well versed in the

---

[1]While this is good practice for all clinicians, it is specifically required for psychologists by the Specialty Guidelines for Forensic Psychologists (Committee on Ethical Guidelines for Forensic Psychologists, 1991). The Specialty Guidelines advise psychologists to properly inform clients about the possible use of information from the therapy relationship in a legal context as soon as it becomes clear that the information may be used in such a context.

type of law related to your case. You may need to find associates in the community who understand the informal rules of professional conduct within the community. If appropriate, consult with your employers and seek out their support for your stance.

Rules versus Fairness

Clinicians often see legal processes as rigid and formal. Attorneys view the rules and structure of these processes as necessary to ensure that the process is predictable and fair. Even when procedural justice is fulfilled in a legal sense, clinicians may see the results of certain cases as unfair and blame bad decisions on legal technicalities.

To some extent, the conflict between rules and fairness is illusory. Legal rules are designed to create a fair process. For example, rules about who can present what evidence and how it should be presented may seem to be unduly restrictive to someone who is unfamiliar with legal processes. While an attorney may seem overly compulsive about details, certainly some degree of precision in details is required to ensure fairness. The better a clinician can understand the reasons for the rules, the more likely he will perceive the rules as fair. However, in some cases, legal processes do indeed seem too rigid and formal for the types of problems that need to be resolved.[2]

Once again, the clinician must decide whether to abide by the rules or challenge them. If you decide to challenge some rules in the legal system, we encourage you to challenge them in a manner consistent with the rules of law. That is, find a way to forward your challenge that does not result in showing disrespect for the system. For example, there are ethical standards as well as professional practice guidelines about how to handle a request from the court to release raw psychological test data. One can challenge a court order to release the raw data by seeking to educate the judge about the ethical constraints placed on their release. One can also offer useful alternatives to the court's directive that may help the court to seek out a different path that avoids that ethical

---

[2]In family law and child welfare cases, for example, clinicians may well prefer mediation or other alternative dispute resolution processes that are designed to take relationship and emotional issues fully into account.

tension between the ethical concerns of the clinician and the litigant's right to due process and a fair trial.

As a witness, you may find that you have little control over the process but that nonetheless it is more appropriate and ultimately more constructive toward achieving your long-term goals to cooperate with authorities. Making long-term systemic changes will probably require that you participate more actively in law reform processes.

Facts versus Subjective Meaning

Adjudicative processes require objective criteria to prove the existence of hard facts and to support particular assessments and recommendations. Clinicians have been accused of having difficulty in distinguishing between fact and speculation. While clinicians use objective criteria for psychological and social assessments, they also employ soft information and subjective opinions. *What happened* is important to attorneys, who are seeking truth in an objective sense, while *the meaning that clients attribute* is important in most clinical processes. From an attorney's perspective, this type of orientation can make a clinician a poor investigator and witness.

How comfortable a clinician feels with legal processes depends in part on the theoretical framework she brings to her clinical practice. Clinicians who employ behaviorism define problems and goals in observable behavioral terms. Behaviorism has a strong history of inquiry using experimental designs. This approach fits well with the needs of an adjudicative process. Cognitive approaches to clinical practice also correspond well with the rational thought processes used in legal argument. In contrast, psychoanalytic therapies are based on abstract constructs and have little experimental research to support their validity. This makes it difficult to use psychoanalytic concepts for evidentiary proof. Similarly, clinicians who use a medical model of practice may adjust to traditional legal processes more easily than clinicians who use a more client-centered approach. Using a medical model, the clinician functions as an expert who can provide a specific diagnosis and prescription for treatment. In contrast, clinicians who use a feminist model of practice may have difficulty providing the type of concrete information needed by the courts. For example, a feminist model might encourage the clinician to view her client as an expert in her own life, which results in avoiding the use of labels, diagnosis, or prescribing for the client.[3] Any request for testimony about the client's current functioning against the standard of the DSM-IV-TR (American Psychiatric Association, 2000) may present a dilemma for such clinicians because they do not typically use such concepts and therefore may not be expert in their application to specific client behaviors.

Some types of research fit better than others with adjudicative processes. Adjudicative decision making requires parties to provide proof of particular facts (Albert, 2000). Accordingly, quantitative research that studies the causal relationships between phenomena fits particularly well. In quantitative research, the researcher begins with a hypothesis and designs a study to test the truth or validity of that hypothesis. Statistical analysis can help to identify the specific probability of particular events. In contrast, judges might question the reliability of findings from qualitative research since this type of methodology lacks the basics of generalizability found in experimental designs (e.g., large, random samples, pre- and posttests, control groups). In order for qualitative research to be accepted as persuasive evidence, a clinician needs to be prepared to demonstrate methods for ensuring its reliability and relevance.[4] Interviewers who are trained to conduct qualitative interviews, for example, will know how to ask questions in a way that limits the effects of their biases on the information provided (LeCompte & Schensul, 1999). Arguably, both narrative and anecdotal evidence fit very well with the common law, which is, after all, a series of narratives or stories of what happened to real people.[5]

How a clinician operates in her clinical role need not limit her ability to be an effective witness. Freida, for example, uses an approach to

---

[3]For a more thorough discussion of theories that inform clinical practice, see Corey (2001). The following general definitions are offered for those who are unfamiliar with the theories identified in this section. According to behaviorism, people learn how to act in response to stimuli in their environments. For example, if a person receives positive reinforcement for behaving in a particular manner, that behavior is more likely to be repeated in the future. According to cognitive theory, people do not simply respond automatically to stimuli but rather are able to think, learn, and make conscious choices about how to act. According to psychoanalytic theory, much of human behavior is dependent on unconscious psychological processes, including sexual and aggressive impulses, repressed childhood memories, and irrational personal conflicts. Feminism explores the unique experiences of women and challenges male-oriented assumptions in traditional theories of psychology and social science.

[4]In qualitative research terms, the concept of "trustworthiness" is used to embrace the quantitative concepts of reliability and validity.

[5]Shuman and Sales (1998) provide a useful conceptual framework of how to think about different types of scientific and clinical testimony in light of different standards of evidence.

family therapy that emphasizes the clients' own subjective meanings of their experiences. If Freida is admitted as an expert witness, she is not limited to this perspective. She can also testify about interpretations from her clinical observations and from other objective data she has gathered. Alternatively, Freida could decide she does not want to be a "good witness." Since Freida is not mandated to provide information to the court, she may specifically decide not to gather objective information about her clients in order to discourage anyone from calling her as a witness. If she is called, any information she possesses will be of little value to the adjudicative process.

Conflicting Roles

When an attorney asks a clinician to act as a witness, the role of witness may conflict with other obligations that a clinician has with his client. For example, the clinician may see himself as an advocate for his client, but the attorney is asking him to present information that undermines his client's interests. Similarly, if the clinician is asked to investigate or monitor a client, the clinician will find it difficult to maintain the trust of the client, which is necessary for an effective clinical relationship. The role boundaries involved in such work are often difficult to navigate. This is why understanding the important role-boundary issues between being both a clinician and a witness is critically important.[6]

Given the potential for conflicts between the roles of clinician and witness, clinicians need to decide whether to maintain both roles. When a clinician is called as a witness, she may need to discontinue service and refer the client to another clinician. For example, if Paula sues Freida for malpractice, Freida will likely decide that she can no longer serve the Carveys. However, Freida still has an ethical obligation to ensure that the family has access to proper services. In cases where the clinician is not being sued but is involved in the client's legal situation as a witness, the clinician may need to consult with colleagues as well as the state licensing board to determine the best course of action. It is important to remember that, even when you agree to testify for your client,

---

[6]For an excellent discussion of role distinctions between clinical and forensic functions, see Greenberg and Shuman (1997). Also, consult your profession's ethical standards and professional practice guidelines for guidance about role boundaries.

you may be asked to disclose information about your client that you are not prepared to openly discuss. Despite your best intentions, once you take the stand, your full file is open to scrutiny by the attorneys and the court. It may become part of the public record. Moreover, you may be asked questions that reveal aspects of your client's behavior that were not expected to become public. The bottom line is that any time you decide to take an advocacy position for a therapy client, you may unintentionally do significant damage to your relationship with that client because of the information you may be compelled to reveal once you are on the stand.

One of the most difficult issues faced when acting as a witness is whether to act as an advocate for the client's wishes or as an objective observer (Ashford, Macht, & Mylym, 1987; Gothard, 1989a). In adjudicative proceedings you will be seen as most credible if you present yourself, as well as your advocacy, in an impartial manner. This may sound paradoxical, but we believe that you should present to the court that your understanding of the issues is drawn solely from your client's perspective. You can also talk about how, as a result of this one-sided influence, you have formed specific beliefs about your client and his understanding of the issues. You may also indicate openness to additional information from other information sources that might help to shed light on aspects of your client's situation that were not presented during therapy.

How you present your advocacy is important. You can advocate and still be viewed as open to new information. Such advocacy may increase the court's view of your credibility. There are other forms of advocacy that come across as rigid and righteous. To illustrate, consider a psychiatrist who is known as an advocate for the rights of people with schizophrenia. The physician believes that, with proper medication and supervision, a particular patient will not pose a risk to self or others and should be released from a mental health institution. To make this point in a credible manner, the psychiatrist could say:

"I have diagnosed this patient personally and I have listened to the views of the other mental health professionals who have testified at this hearing. I understand that they are concerned about his history of setting fires. During the past 2 weeks, under my medical supervision, the patient has been cooperative with his medication regimen and his auditory hallucinations have ceased. If he continues to comply with treatment, he will not have the type of hallucinations that prompted his fire-setting conduct in the past."

Contrast this approach with the following:

"The professionals who testified against my patient do not know what they are talking about because they haven't been working with him. This patient's right to autonomy has been violated by keeping him locked up against his will. He poses no threat to anyone and must be allowed to live in the community."

If the psychiatrist shows rigid and righteous bias toward a particular client with schizophrenia, her testimony will be given little weight. She may even severely damage her own professional reputation.

Most ethically interesting and morally challenging is when you are asked to provide testimony that is contrary to your client's interest. When you are asked to provide such testimony, you may feel as though it is a betrayal of your client. You and your client should discuss his feelings about your upcoming testimony. It may be useful to talk about different scenarios that may play out in court, such as hostile examination that reveals testimony that was never intended to be divulged. Exploring these possible situations with your client may help to clarify in your own mind the appropriateness of your agreement to testify.

For example, Freida feels sympathetic toward Paula and struggles with how she could say anything that could put Paula's position at risk. In some situations, your testimony may be in the client's or community's best interests, even though it is not the type of information the client wants to hear. In contrast to purely adjudicative proceedings, in political or legislative proceedings acting as an advocate can be highly appropriate and may even be the normal expectation.

Dilemmas may arise because of conflicting legal and ethical obligations. The code of ethics for your professional association may censure what you are asked to do as a witness. Suppose, for example, a psychological association has a policy supporting a woman's right to choice regarding abortion. Would it be ethical for a psychologist to provide evidence in a case that supports a pro-life perspective? In other circumstances, a clinician may receive an unethical request from an attorney. Lori could ask Evelyn not to report certain information that hurts her client's case. Although Lori is not specifically asking Evelyn to lie, does

Lori have an obligation to report full and frank information? Such dilemmas have no easy answer. They depend upon the clinician's role and professional obligations. If Evelyn were hired by Philip's attorney to do an assessment, her obligations under attorney work product rules would be different from those if she were appointed by the court or hired jointly by Philip and Paula. (For further discussion, see Chapter 7.) If Philip rather than Philip's attorney hired Evelyn, her obligations would also be different.

Rights versus Therapeutic Goals

Typically attorneys are concerned about the legal rights of individuals, whereas clinicians are concerned about social and psychological goals (Harris, Qualls, Harris, & Harris, 2000). Some attorneys have prior education and background in mental health or social work, while some law schools provide courses to create sensitivities to community issues and to develop counseling skills (Binder, Bergman, & Price, 1991). Still, many clinicians believe attorneys focus on rights while taking insufficient account of the emotional effects and broader social impacts that legal cases have on individual clients and their families.

Both clinicians and attorneys believe people should take responsibility for their actions. This principle often manifests differently in the preferred methods of the two professions. The foci of the criminal justice system, for example, are retribution and protection of the public. If someone commits a wrong, justice demands that she be punished. Punishment is also used to deter or prevent further criminal acts. Although rehabilitation plays a role in the system, clinicians often note that the rehabilitation aspect of the system is undervalued. If a clinician believes that an individual is in need of therapeutic treatment or has been deprived of a supportive social environment, she may sympathize with the individual. To advance these concerns in legal processes, a clinician may need to translate them into language that fits in a legal framework. Sam might believe Philip's abusive behavior is the result of mistreatment in his own upbringing. The law does not view disadvantages in one's upbringing as an excuse for behavior. However, Sam could present information at the sentencing phase of a criminal trial that suggests how a therapeutic response could be used to prevent Philip from being abusive in the future. This type of argument must be based on research that demonstrates the effectiveness of the prescribed intervention. Unfortunately, there is little research support for the efficacy of many treatment interventions despite the fact that clinicians continue to employ such unproven strategies.

Lack of Respect

The final type of potential conflict stems from disrespect between attorneys and clinicians. Lack of respect may result from ignorance or negative experiences with individuals in the other profession. For instance, Lori may have had difficulty with a psychiatrist as a witness in a prior case. Evelyn may view attorneys as "hired guns," determined to win at all costs. Resentment and disrespect often result from differences in status and pay between the two types of professions. Disrespectful behavior is sometimes an intentional strategy, such as when an attorney uses intimidation to discredit a witness, "forgets" to provide the clinician with significant information, or sends threatening letters. Ethically both attorneys and clinicians have a duty to show respect for other professionals and in fact, for all individuals. Despite negative clichés about attorneys, they typically behave ethically.

Extreme cases may require that you report unethical behavior to the law society. However, your customary mental health or social work strategies can be used to defuse most situations: active listening, time-outs, identifying mutual concerns, constructive confrontation, nonjudgmental assertiveness, meeting the attorney halfway, and using "I" statements to indicate what type of treatment you prefer. This does not mean providing therapy to the attorney—regardless of whether the attorney could use it.

Consider an attorney who shows little respect for social workers. The attorney may see social workers as well-meaning and charitable but as having little training or expertise. If the social worker becomes defensive and loses his temper with the attorney, this behavior reinforces the attorney's stereotype. If the social worker tunes in to the reasons for the attorney's treatment, then the social worker may be able to confront the attorney in a constructive manner. For example, the attorney may not know the extent of the social worker's knowledge and skills, or may believe anyone can practice social work. The social worker can address these concerns by providing information about his educational background, standards of practice, specific areas of expertise, and the science behind social work. Being certified or registered by a social work association can raise the social worker's standing with legal professionals. Having your own attorney present will also reduce the likelihood of being treated with disrespect.

Disrespect may also stem from differences in the ethics of the two professions. Attorneys have an ethical obligation to advance their clients' cause resolutely. A clinician may question how an attorney could defend people who have committed criminal acts. To see this issue from the attorney's perspective, the clinician needs to consider the "right to an attorney" and "presumption of innocence" as essential components of a fair legal process.

CONCLUSION

Knowledge and experience will help to reduce anxiety and provide a feeling of greater control when you are involved in legal proceedings. In some situations, acting as a witness will be smooth and straightforward. Awareness of potentially difficult situations is the first step in preparing for worst-case scenarios. If you have had negative experiences with legal processes, you need to ensure that they do not interfere with your ability to be effective as a witness in the future. If you view legal processes positively, then you will have an easier time working in this context. If you have taken the time to reflect on the legal system and still do not respect its processes, rules, or values, then your participation will be more difficult. While you may decide to take a stance or advocate for change, choose your battles wisely.

Chapter 3

First Contact

Assume you are going about your clinical practice, minding your own business. A client calls and wants to talk with you about his impending legal proceeding and his expectations that you will testify for him. Perhaps an attorney calls to inform you about a complaint soon to be filed against you. Or, perhaps, an officer from the sheriff's department knocks on your door during a therapy session. Standing there, in full uniform, gun in holster, she hands you a subpoena and asks you to sign a form acknowledging service. You sign the acknowledgment and before you can ask what the subpoena is for, the officer walks out of the building. You turn around and see your client, eyes popping out of his head, wondering what you could possibly have done.

Take a deep breath and don't worry about any of these circumstances. This chapter describes how to respond to initial contacts with "legal situations" where you have been working with clients on a voluntary basis. How you react at these initial stages can dramatically affect whether and how you will be involved in any subsequent proceedings.

CONTACTED TO BE A WITNESS OR TO PROVIDE INFORMATION

When an attorney calls or writes about a legal proceeding, many clinicians feel caught off guard. Having a standard procedure in place for dealing with contacts from attorneys will help you to feel prepared and not have that "Oh, my gosh, what do I do now?" feeling.

The first step is to have a written policy established. This written policy should include who in your practice or agency should respond in writing to the initial legal contact. You should also have determined who should be consulted. You may wish to involve your practice or agency attorney as well as colleagues and staff. It is critical that the written policy explain issues of confidentiality pertaining to the legal contact as well as issues about client–clinician privilege. You may also describe how you will handle the exchange of information, anticipated affidavits, declarations, depositions, and testimony. Included in this initial policy statement should also be reference to payment issues. We strongly advise that any policy statement written for your practice or agency be thoroughly reviewed by your attorney.

When an attorney contacts you, you need to gather certain information before providing any information to the attorney.[1] Ask the attorney:

- Which person do you represent?
- How did you get my name?
- What is the nature of the concerns or proceedings?
- What information do you want?
- Why is this information needed?
- How do you want to get this information (e.g., written report, telephone meeting, meeting in person)?
- What is the time frame for the request?

During the initial contact you do not need to give the attorney any commitments on these issues or even admit that the person referred to is your client. Instead, say something like this:

"The policy of my agency requires that I first gather information about the nature of your request. Out of respect for client confidentiality, I cannot tell you whether this person is a client of this

---

[1]As a standard precaution, never speak to anyone in detail until you are sure the person is who he says he is. Law societies have registries of attorneys if you want to call to verify whether the person is a licensed attorney. At the very least, check a telephone directory for the accuracy of the telephone number and address provided. Although these precautions may sound paranoid, anyone could call you and claim to be someone entitled to your client's information. In fact, the caller could be an ex-spouse who is stalking your client, a family member, a nosy neighbor, or whoever.

agency. If the person is a client, I will need to speak with her and obtain a written release for confidential information. I will call you by [date] to let you know whether I have consent to speak with you. If I do not have a consent, then either this person is not a client or the person is a client but refused consent to speak with you."

The attorney may be frustrated that you are not immediately providing the information he is seeking. Reassure him that you need to understand the request and follow the ethical rules of your profession before releasing any information, including whether or not the individual is a client. Rather than stressing that you want to be cooperative, you may wish to emphasize that your responsibility is to those people who use your clinical services and that you will take the ethically appropriate and legally necessary steps to properly respond to the attorney's request. You may also want to provide the attorney with your preferred time frame, suggesting that you will provide some sort of response to his initial inquiry by a specified date. For example: "I will consider your request for information and, upon receipt of the signed release of information form you have in your possession, I will make the necessary calls and call you back within 5 working days."

If the attorney tries to pressure you into responding immediately, resist getting into discussions before you have the proper releases and you have discussed with your client the information you intend to share with the attorney. It is common for clinicians to feel a sense of wanting to help. This is often part of why we went into a helping profession. So, when an attorney or a judge asks for information that appears helpful to your client, there is a tendency to want to help by disclosing the information. However, releasing information because you wanted to help *before* you have the proper releases and a solid understanding with your client of what will be disclosed may injure the therapeutic relationship. It may result in overstepping ethical boundaries that are in place to protect your client's right to privacy. So, the moral of the story is *never* disclose any information about your client until you have all the proper releases signed and in your file.

Do not be surprised if the attorney attempts to engage you in conversation. His job is to obtain the needed information. However, your job is to provide the information only upon proper release. You do not want to get caught off guard by the attorney's questions. Returning to our case example, Lori might ask Evelyn whether she followed her usual and customary procedures for assessing the Carveys. If Evelyn answers, "No," she may be challenged on the basis of bias, alleging that she varied from her usual and customary procedures without any convincing reason to do so. Or, if the variations from standard procedures are changes unsupported by research or community standards, she might face a complaint to the licensing board and/or a civil suit for malpractice (which we will discuss in detail in Chapter 9).

It is important that you understand the legal implications of the issues involved in the case. It is also important that you understand the limits and boundaries of your testimonial competencies. As long as you stay within what you know and what you are professionally permitted to testify about, you will have little difficulty in the legal system. Once you step outside the boundaries of your testimonial competencies, then you are vulnerable to ethical and legal challenges. The key is *always* to consult with colleagues and your attorney if you have any concerns about contact from a lawyer or your potential appearance as a witness in a legal proceeding.

It is also important to know what should and should not be discussed over the telephone. There are times when an attorney may call to ask your opinion about an issue about which you have knowledge, although you are not part of his case. Once you provide that information, the attorney may present it in some form in his legal case. This might result in your being called to testify about your statement even though you made the statement off-the-cuff and assumed it was not for public consumption. Be certain with the person on the other end of the telephone line that you will not discuss aspects of a case without a clear understanding of how the information will be used. Similarly, you may need to ask clearly at the beginning of a conversation whether the attorney is recording the phone call or taking contemporaneous notes. Knowing whether the attorney is taking notes or recording your conversation should help alert you to what you are able to say and how it may be used. You should not consent to his recording the call, and you should not continue your participation in the telephone call.

If the attorney expresses urgency in her request, ask about the nature of the urgency. To the extent that you understand the urgency, you may be better able to respond. If there is an upcoming court date, there may be the possibility of a continuance. Even if the urgency is caused by the attorney's procrastination or misuse of time in handling a case, you and your client's interests may still be best served by being cooperative.

Sometimes an attorney will request information from your file. In one scenario, Philip's attorney, Lori, may request copies of Freida's notes and assessments in her efforts to file a motion to increase Philip's times for visitation with his daughter, Debra. As the family therapist, Freida needs to obtain written releases from both parents. If either parent refuses to provide a release, Freida may be ethically and legally bound not to release the information unless a subpoena or court order requires her to do so (see "Confidentiality, Privilege, and Exceptions," below). In addition to the client, there may be others you need to consult before providing information to an attorney. If you are working in an agency context, you may need to consult your supervisor, the director of the program, or the agency's attorney. If you are a member of a professional organization, you may want to consult with the association.

In our ongoing example, Michael may have been contacted first by Paula's attorney as a potential witness. As a professional courtesy, Lori should ask Paula's attorney for permission to speak with Michael, the mediator. If Lori calls Michael directly, Michael should consult with Paula's attorney to decide whether he should meet with Lori and, if so, how. There is no prohibition against speaking with attorneys for both parties to a dispute, so long as issues of confidence and privilege are clearly discussed up front. These issues should be reduced to writing in the form of a letter sent to all parties to ensure that all sides understand the rules about such conversations. During the conversation, Michael should take notes about the discussion. Upon completion of such conversations, Michael would be wise to write a summary of his notes taken during the conversation and either file the notes for future reference or, if allowed, forward a letter to both attorneys summarizing his understanding of the outcome of the conversation. In this way Michael may avoid getting caught in a crossfire between attorneys who might disagree about the content and meaning of the conversation.

It may be the client who asks for information that could be used in a legal proceeding. If the information is about the client, then the client generally has a right to those records. If you are concerned that your actions may be called into question at a legal proceeding, then you should contact your own attorney.

There are two components to this scenario. The first is the legal and ethical responsibility you have to release records upon your client's proper written authorization. The second is the treatment issue of how the information will be released and what information will be released.

It may be wise to talk with your client about the purpose of releasing the information and how best to release the information in a manner that may preserve some protection for your client–therapist relationship. It also may be useful to talk with your attorney about crafting a release statement, that is, a statement that clearly defines and limits what information will be permitted to be released from the file. There are important legal issues about confidentiality involved in your decision to release the file. There may be ways to release some information while protecting other information. Your attorney and your client's attorney may wish to talk with each other in an attempt to frame a written consent to release that limits both the information to be released and the persons to whom the information may be released.

Providing the requested information may help your client resolve a problem without going to court. In the Carvey's case, Freida may have information that the parties could consider in order to negotiate a separation agreement. Withholding this information may cause more difficulties for all concerned, and, if all releases are properly signed and executed, it may be unethical and illegal for Freida to withhold such information.

Do Witnesses Need Legal Representation?

Ordinarily, when a person is acting as a witness, he does not need his own attorney. As a clinician with professional obligations and standards, you may want to consult an attorney for advice about confidentiality issues, ethical dilemmas, or information about how best to present evidence. There are continuing education workshops presented frequently around the country that focus on ethical behavior. Among these workshops are presentations about clinical treatment ethics, forensic treatment ethics, and forensic evaluation ethics.

When an attorney is acting for a client and contacts you as a potential witness, that attorney does not represent you in the proceedings. The attorney calling you as a witness may be a "friendly attorney," meaning a lawyer representing interests that are generally consistent with your own. However, that attorney's responsibility is to his client and not to you. He may be unable to provide you with any advice because of the potential for a conflict of interest to emerge. That conflict would be providing legal advice to you while representing your client. No matter how "friendly" your client's attorney may be, he is not your advocate and may be unable to protect you. To illustrate, consider a request from Lori to Freida to act as a witness in support of Philip's application for visitation. If Freida had information that supported this motion, then Lori may be considered to be a friendly attorney from Freida's perspective. Paula's attorney would be considered an opposing attorney, since he represents Paula's interests, which are adverse to Philip's interests.

Although the friendly attorney does not represent you, the attorney may offer guidance and information to help you in your role as a witness to the extent that it helps his client. The information that you have to offer as evidence is information that generally supports the friendly attorney's case. Often the attorney's focus is on winning his case, not on having truth revealed. Your clinical truth may, in some ways, support his case. It will likely be that he will want to encourage you to discuss that aspect of your case. However, you will have an ethical responsibility to present a fair and unbiased representation of your work, not just the aspects that favor the attorney's case. As such, aspects of your testimony may place you at odds with the attorney, who may discourage you from testifying about the full picture. This is when you must examine yourself and whom you choose to be as a witness. Are you someone who advocates for a client or someone who advocates for the truth of your experience? When they are the same, this is not a problem. When they are different, the moral and ethical challenge is to be cognizant of the dilemma and consider what is professionally responsible behavior.[2] To illustrate, consider the following example:

> Evelyn, the custody evaluator, conducts an evaluation that leads her to conclude that Debra's primary residence should be with her mother, Paula, but that both Paula and Philip should share parental decision-making responsibility (i.e., joint legal custody). Lori, Philip's lawyer, asks Evelyn to stress information that Philip is a good father and minimize her findings that favor Paula providing the primary residence for Debra. Although Evelyn does not want to embarrass Philip with her testimony, her professional obligation is to provide both strengths and limitations of his parenting ability.

---

[2]See Lavin and Sales (1998) for a discussion of the moral foundations of expert witness testimony.

You need to be aware of the limits of this attorney's support. Parts of your information and beliefs may go against the attorney's case. Attorneys are generally restricted from challenging or discrediting their own witnesses during a hearing. During preparation stages, however, you and the attorney may not know whether your evidence will be advantageous to the attorney's case and whether you will ultimately be called as a witness. You may also be hesitant to disclose information to a "friendly attorney" that could be used against you at a subsequent hearing. If the attorney were your own attorney, you could feel free to disclose this information because your conversations with your own attorney are protected by confidentiality; in fact, your attorney needs full disclosure in order to advise you properly. If you disclose controversial information to a friendly attorney, you do not have the same degree of control in keeping information confidential. In fact, you may have *no* control over how that information is subsequently used in litigation. It is always wise to have the friendly attorney provide *in writing* an explanation of how your treatment information is to be used. In this way you and your client can craft a release of information that may narrowly define what information will be released and how it is to be used. Since state laws may differ on this point, it may be useful to consult both your attorney as well as the attorney for your professional association.

A CLIENT COMPLAINS

When a client complains, the clinician may feel threatened or defensive. When threatened, our natural instinct may be to fight or flee. However, aggressively confronting a client, denying an allegation, or running for cover is more likely to anger the client, resulting in an exacerbation of the problem rather than its resolution. Even if you have practiced in an ethical and competent manner, a complaint may be made. Sometimes a complaint is the result of an angry parent in a custody battle who is seeking a target for his or her anger resulting from loss of custody.[3] Sometimes a complaint is the result of a misunderstanding. Sometimes a complaint is the result of sheer vengeance.

---

[3]See Kirkland and Kirkland (2001) regarding child custody complaints to licensing boards and suggestions for anticipatory defensive steps to protect the evaluator.

Other times, a complaint is the result of poor judgment on the part of the clinician.

If a client complains directly to you, the best approach is to talk with the client about the concerns. Conflict resolution and negotiation skills are important to use in such situations (Barsky, 2000). People often respond best when they feel that their story has been heard. Once you have demonstrated that you have listened to the other's concerns, that person may be more open to listening to you (Mayer, 2000). The idea of "seeking first to understand and then be understood" is a useful framework in approaching a client who complains directly to you.

Many cases that end up in court could have been resolved much earlier if the parties had just tried to talk about their concerns in an informal and civilized manner. Calling an attorney at this stage is advisable if a specific action such as a complaint or lawsuit has been initiated. Calling an attorney is also advisable if the client has suffered harm. Otherwise, you are probably better off to invite the client to speak with you to try to work things out. Many complaints arise out of miscommunication. Many requests are calls for information or listening. Use your clinical therapeutic skills: meet face-to-face, be supportive, explore the client's concerns, recognize the feelings of a client who believes she has been wronged, listen and demonstrate that you understand (Barsky, 2000; Mayer, 2000). If the client is asking for a remedy, find out what that is. It may be an explanation or an apology. She may want her complaint to be heard and acknowledged by a supervisor or person in authority.

If you have *any* doubts about how to respond, consult with a supervisor, a colleague, your insurance company, or your professional association. Admissions or offers to remedy can incur significant legal consequences. They might even void an insurance policy. The point is not to offer any remedy before you have explored the legal consequences of your remedy.

If an attorney calls or writes regarding a complaint directed against you, do not answer the complaint until you have spoken with your supervisor, attorney, insurance adjuster, and/or professional association for advice:

> "As you can understand, I cannot speak with you about these concerns. I will have my attorney contact you."

Once you receive notice of a formal complaint against you, either in the form of a licensing board complaint or a law suit, immediately contact your professional liability insurance company where you or your agency hold a policy. (You *are* insured, right?)

If a client has a complaint against another practitioner, you may be asked to help your client talk with the alleged offending professional. Although you may feel a strong allegiance to help your client, you need to ask if the support being sought is within your role as a treating therapist. It is easy to get caught up in the client's need for support and guidance. It is also easy to get pulled into something that is outside the realm of your professional competence or role. This is a way to step into the client's conflict rather than staying within your properly defined role as a clinician.

The more you step outside your role or boundaries as treating clinician, the greater the likelihood that you will become part of the conflict (Reamer, 2001). Once outside your properly defined role, you may become the target of a complaint by the other professional, who would argue that you placed yourself in a dual-role situation with the complaining client. It may be appropriate to refer the client to another professional who can assist in resolving the conflict. However, never choose to be that person who works at resolving the conflict while you are also the client's clinician (Barsky, 2000; Mayer, 2000).

If a client makes allegations against you, then legal representation is imperative. (See Chapter 9 on malpractice.) Charges against Michael for unauthorized practice of law or a civil lawsuit against Freida for malpractice are clear examples calling for the use of attorneys. Other situations are not as clear-cut. For example, Sam could be involved in the inquest concerning a child's death. He may not know that his conduct is being questioned and that there might be legal consequences for his participation in the inquest. Err on the side of caution, and consult an attorney as soon as you become aware that you are involved in an aspect of another person's legal dispute.

SELECTING AN ATTORNEY

Identifying and becoming acquainted with an attorney before trouble arises is better than waiting until you are subpoenaed or sued. By developing a positive rapport, you will know that you have a trusted confidant to turn to when you have the need for legal advice. Ideally your agency or private practice has an attorney who is familiar with your type of work on permanent retainer for consultation. We suggest developing a relationship with a private attorney as well. In this way you will have an attorney who is *always* your advocate and independent of any possible conflicts that might arise if you share the same attorney as your agency or practice.

If you do not already have an attorney in mind, there are several sources to consider. The board of directors of your agency might include an attorney whom you could consult. If you and your agency have conflicting interests in a legal proceeding, you may need a different attorney from the one used by the agency. You may have used an attorney to help set up your practice—to incorporate, to develop service agreements, and so on. If you are involved in a particular legal proceeding, you may want to retain the services of an attorney with special expertise (e.g., malpractice litigation, criminal law, or mental health proceedings). A coprofessional could provide you with a referral to an attorney she trusts, or your state professional association may have knowledge of attorneys who have practiced in your field. Finally, state or local bar associations in some jurisdictions offer attorney referral services where you are provided with the names and telephone numbers of a few attorneys in your area. Some of these services may provide you with a free half-hour consultation to help you decide whether to retain that attorney. Financial arrangements for the initial meeting should be discussed during the initial phone consultation.

There is no general right to legal counsel for witnesses involved in legal proceedings. If you are the defendant in a criminal trial, you have a right to counsel. Accordingly, a publicly funded legal aid organization will pay all or part of the fees of an attorney for a person who is accused of a criminal offence and does not have the means to pay for the attorney. The rules for legal aid vary across jurisdictions in relation to what other types of cases legal aid will cover, but they are generally quite limited. If you have professional insurance, the insurance company may provide for legal representation in cases where you are a party to a legal proceeding but not where you are just a witness.[4] Professional associations may have attorney referral information.

---

[4]Many professional liability insurance companies provide separate coverage funds for civil litigation and for defense of licensing board complaints. These funds are typically limited and subject to certain conditions. Check your policy to ensure that you are covered for each possible occurrence, including an adequate level of coverage.

Ideally you will have lots of lead time and the freedom to select an attorney who can provide you with the services you need. Do not be shy about asking for information before retaining an attorney. Focus on information that indicates the attorney's competence: length, quality, and relevance of experience; specialized training; reputation; and skills for resolving cases in negotiation (including "collaborative lawyering") versus litigation. Consider pragmatic concerns such as time and money. An attorney with a great reputation may charge more than you can afford and may have little time for low-profile cases. You want an attorney who will pay due consideration to your case. Most attorneys work on an hourly basis. Ask what the hourly rate is, as well as an estimate of the expected time for completion of the case. The attorney may ask for a payment up front as a retainer. Let the attorney know how often you wish to be billed or inquire as to the law firm's billing cycle. Let your attorney know that you want him to check with you before incurring additional legal costs. Finally, ensure that the attorney does not have any conflict of interest (such as also representing your client).[5]

CONFIDENTIALITY, PRIVILEGE, AND EXCEPTIONS

Although the issues of confidentiality and privilege are straightforward in most cases, conflict and controversy do have the potential to arise. Laws, ethical codes, and agency policies are still evolving, particularly with respect to domestic violence, child maltreatment, sexual abuse, and other forms of domestic unrest. In this section, we first discuss the general principles of confidentiality and privilege. We then describe four exceptions to those principles: duties to report; consent to disclose; access to information legislation; and compelling a clinician to disclose.

The obligation for clinicians to maintain confidentiality has several sources. As an ethical principle, most codes of professional conduct prescribe confidentiality and its limits. As a clinical strategy, confidentiality is offered to clients to build a safe environment in which to talk openly about personal, relationship, workplace, or family concerns, knowing

---

[5]As a customary procedure, most law firms conduct an in-office search to ensure there is no conflict of interest, prior to accepting a new case.

that no one else will ever know what is discussed behind the closed doors of therapy. In most therapeutic models a client's trust is considered essential for effective collaborative work. As a legal obligation, the statutes and policies governing private practice as well as clinical agencies generally require the protection of a client's right to privacy. As a contractual obligation, confidentiality is usually a key component of the clinician–client contract for work, whether that contract is written, oral, or implied.[6]

Attorneys also value confidentiality. In fact, confidentiality of information gathered within an attorney–client relationship is well protected by law. Conflict between clinicians and attorneys arises, however, when attorneys challenge the confidentiality of the clinician–client relationship in order to further their case in legal proceedings. In some states clinician–client confidentiality is an absolute right, while in other states the right to confidentiality can be legally challenged (Saltzman & Furman, 1999).

Legal processes may require the disclosure of information to facilitate the search for truth and justice. In addition, most cases are open to the public to ensure accountability. Clinicians view forced disclosure and public access to information as infringements on a client's right to confidentiality as well as a serious threat to the integrity of the therapeutic relationship. Clinicians need to discuss the limits of confidentiality with their clients from the outset of their work together. Sometimes a clinician–client relationship can be maintained even after a clinician provides disturbing testimony against a client if the release to disclose information is properly crafted to limit what can be said and to whom. In other cases, the client will lose trust, become angry, or rebel against the clinician. More empirical research is required to explore the actual impact of forced disclosure (e.g., such matters as the impact on clinician–client relationships following disclosure and whether laws that favor disclosure increase client reluctance to seek clinical help in the future).

Disclosure in legal proceedings does not necessarily conflict with the interests of clinicians. Hearings may be viewed as a form of enforc-

---

[6]From a legal perspective, preferred practice suggests you should always have a signed informed-consent contract specifying the limitations of confidentiality, as well as a description of privilege.

ing accountability. Accountability advances the interests of both clients and the public. In child protection proceedings, the court would review Sam's work to ensure that his investigation was thorough and that he followed proper standards of practice. Sometimes clinicians are too quick to argue for confidentiality, perhaps seeing it as an absolute value or using it defensively to protect their own interests.

Privilege is a legal concept related to the principle of confidentiality. Where privilege is recognized, information gained during the course of certain professional relationships is protected from having to be disclosed in court or other legal processes. Privilege is intended to preserve communications that were not intended to be disclosed to others. Privilege may be prescribed by legislation or recognized by common law.[7] Common law, for example, recognizes the attorney–client privilege. With few exceptions, an attorney cannot disclose communications between the attorney and her client without consent of the client. Family law legislation in some jurisdictions recognizes "closed mediation," which protects information from being disclosed during the course of mediation.[8] Certain medical and adoption records may also be protected by legislation. Some jurisdictions in the United States have legislation that grants privilege to communications with certain regulated clinical professionals. Other states do not have privilege created by statute, though there may be limited privilege at common law. Privilege exists only for information intended to be kept confidential. For example, neither Paula nor Philip could claim privilege for information gathered by Evelyn if both parties initially agreed that Evelyn's evaluation would be used in court. In fact, if Evelyn is a court-appointed expert, Evelyn's client is the court rather than the parents. There is no legal relationship between Evelyn and the parents. The legal relationship is between Evelyn and the court, meaning that issues of privilege and confidence are between the court and the evaluator.[9]

Issues related to privilege can also arise when one attorney hires

---

[7]"Common law" refers to law derived from cases decided by judges, as opposed to statutes passed by the legislature.

[8]For a discussion of proposed uniform legislation on confidentiality in mediation, see the Association for Conflict Resolution web site at *http://www.acresolution.org*.

[9]For further discussion of this important distinction, see CEGFP (1991), Gould (1998), Gould and Bell (2000), Gould and Stahl (2000), and Greenberg and Shuman (1997).

you to help with a case and then the attorney for the other side calls. This situation has several interesting aspects to it. For example, you may not be allowed to acknowledge to the second attorney that the first attorney has retained you. Alternatively, you may be allowed to acknowledge that you have been retained but not allowed to talk about the focus of your work. "Attorney work product privilege" is a legal concept that protects any and all information discussed between the attorney and you as an expert who is assisting with preparation for a case. Until the attorney decides to reveal your participation, you may not be allowed to talk with anyone about your involvement. It is essential that you and the attorney who hired you are clear about what can and cannot be discussed with others *before* you talk with anyone else!

Police and Duties to Report

As a general rule, clinicians have no duty to report illegal behavior to police when it is discussed within the privacy of therapy. If, during family therapy, Paula said that she used to sell cocaine because she needed the money, Freida would not have to report Paula. There are many exceptions to this "general rule." For example, in the interests of protecting children from maltreatment, the laws in most jurisdictions require clinicians to report suspicions and actual incidents of abuse and neglect to the police or to child protection authorities.[10] Probation and parole officers are obliged to act on breaches of probation and to report certain crimes. Health professionals in some jurisdictions have a duty to trace partners of patients with certain communicable diseases such as HIV, and they may also have a duty to report abuse toward the elderly or people with disabilities.

Another exception arises when a clinician learns of information where there is clear danger of harm (e.g., a client intends to shoot another person or plans to commit suicide). Codes of ethics generally permit breaches of confidentiality to protect an identifiable and foreseeable victim. American case law suggests that clinicians have an affirmative duty to warn (*Tarasoff v. Regents of University of California*, 1976) as well

---

[10]Check your local state statutes, as well as the code of ethics for your professional association, for your specific reporting obligations regarding actual or suspected abuse of children, elderly adults, and people with disabilities.

as a duty to protect.[11] If you are unsure whether the level of risk in a particular case triggers either duty, consult an attorney. Possible clinician responses include, but are not limited to:

- Counseling the client to deal with the underlying cause of the risk.
- Warning the potential victim.
- Referring the client for a second-level assessment.
- Starting civil commitment proceedings.
- Calling the police.

Each situation will require its own response. The clinician must weigh respect for the individual's right to autonomy against the interests in preventing harm. Even if there is no legal duty to prevent harm, erring on the side of life and safety is generally preferred (Parsons, 2000; Reamer, 2001). On the other hand, clinicians must be careful not to overanticipate danger as a means of covering themselves against lawsuits—at the peril of completely diminishing client rights to confidentiality.

When a clinician acts to prevent child maltreatment or other foreseeable harm, the rights to confidentiality and privilege are not completely forfeited. The clinician should release only information necessary to prevent the harm. Once authorities have gathered information from a clinician, they may try to use that information in future proceedings. The issue of what information can be used in court is separate from the issue of what information has to be reported to police or to the potential victim to prevent harm (Dickson, 1995; Saltzman & Furman, 1999). For instance, if Michael told police that Philip planned to abduct Debra, the police could act on this information in order to ensure Debra's safety (e.g., stake out Debra's day care center to ensure that Philip does not try to abduct Debra). If Philip showed up at the day care center and tried to take Debra, the police could arrest Philip and charge him with attempted abduction. At trial, if Michael were called to testify

---

[11]In Tarasoff, the California Supreme Court ruled that a therapist has a duty to warn known potential victims about threats made by dangerous patients. This is commonly referred to as Tarasoff I. Tarasoff II concluded that therapists have a duty to protect (rather than just a duty to warn) innocent parties about potentially dangerous clients. Issuing a warning is included as an option under the duty to protect (see also American Psychological Association, 1995; National Association of Social Workers, 2001).

about Philip's abduction plans, Philip's lawyer could claim privilege even though Michael had reported the plans to the police. The court would have to determine whether to breach the privilege, weighing concerns about protecting confidential mediation relationships against the need for evidence to ensure a just decision by the court.

In some child abuse and sexual assault investigations, police and clinicians conduct joint interviews. This approach allows police to gather evidence and clinicians to offer therapeutic help in a coordinated process.[12] The information received by police in a joint interview with a clinician would not be privileged. The police and clinical agencies should have a protocol for joint work, specifying who has access to what information held by the other organization. The protocols may even require police to use a warrant or subpoena from the court for formal production of the clinician's files.

If the police contact you during a criminal investigation, you should generally refrain from discussing confidential information unless there is a subpoena or an order from the court (discussed below). Information you share with the police may be provided to the district attorney (the prosecution attorneys). The district attorney may enter this information into the court record. Information obtained by the district attorney may also be subject to disclosure to the accused, so that his attorney can prepare for trial. You should cooperate with the police as necessary to prevent the occurrence of significant harm (particularly, danger to people) while at the same time maintaining a watchful eye on your ethical responsibilities to your clients.

Finally, a duty to disclose information may arise if a clinician knows of information that could prevent a miscarriage of justice. Unless a clinician is a probation officer or other officer of the court, there is no legal obligation to report in this circumstance, but one may be ethically justified in breaching confidentiality. Consider if Michael were not called to court but had material evidence that could prevent a criminal conviction against Philip. The clinician faces an ethical dilemma—does his obligation to confidentiality override the interest in avoiding a wrongful conviction? There is no clear law on this matter. A clinician

---

[12]The use of cooperative interviews serving dual purposes is controversial. An investigative interview follows a different path than a therapeutic interview. When the two are used together, especially with young children, there is an increased likelihood that the information obtained from the young child is influenced by the context of the interview process. This may reduce the usefulness of the child's information for legal or forensic evaluation purposes (Ceci & Bruck, 1995; Poole & Lamb, 1998).

faced with this issue should refer to her agency's policies and consult an attorney and her professional association.

Consent to Disclose Information

Where confidentiality and privilege are recognized, these rights are generally the client's rather than the clinician's. As a result, a client may consent to the release of confidential information or waive his right to privilege. The clinician cannot argue for confidentiality or privilege if the client has agreed to disclosure unless there is legislation specifically giving privilege to the clinician.

The preferred practice for obtaining permission to release information specifies that the consent be informed, voluntary, signed, dated, and specific. To ensure that consent is informed, you should explain the consent in plain language, giving your client the opportunity to ask questions. If there are any questions about the client's mental capacity, explore the client's ability to understand the nature of the agreement. Mental capacity can be affected by mental illnesses, substance abuse, or the stress of legal proceedings. If there are legal complexities or questions about the client's capacity, consider providing the client access to legal advice before signing. To test for voluntariness of the consent explore your client's reasons for signing the consent and the possibility of coercion or pressure. Ensure that the consent form is signed by someone who is legally authorized to provide consent. Both Philip and Paula would need to sign a consent form in order for Freida to release information about the couple's therapy. For information about Debra, her clinician would need to know who had legal custody. In terms of specific details in the release, the consent should include the scope of the information to be released, by whom, to whom, for what purposes, and over what period of time. An oral consent may be required for pragmatic reasons such as time constraints. In that case, you should note the consent in your client records.[13]

---

[13]In cases where an individual is referred for evaluation or therapy by a third party such as the court, the referred individual might be advised to review the informed consent with his attorney. An individual referred by the court may be unable to provide voluntary informed consent in the clinician's office. The rationale is that signing the consent in the office may be the result of coercion—the signing party might feel compelled to sign the consent in order to please the needs of the court. Allowing the signing of consent to occur between the party and his attorney may avoid such appearance of coercion, though the clinician should recognize that the client may still feel he is attending therapy or the evaluation under some pressure.

In cases where privilege is requested, the request must come from the client or the client's lawyer, not from you as the clinician. If you are called to testify, find out ahead of time whether the client intends to claim or to waive her right to privilege. In certain instances a client is deemed to have waived her right to privilege, such as when a client introduces confidential information into a hearing or when a client sues her clinician. This allows the clinician to respond to statements or allegations made by the client concerning the therapeutic process. For example, if Philip based his defense on having progressed well in therapy, the clinician could be asked for her evaluation. If Paula sued Michael for malpractice, she could not deny his right to respond by claiming that the information was privileged. It is always safer to obtain written consent before providing testimony. If that is not possible, then ask to obtain verbal consent on the record prior to beginning testimony. If you are unable to obtain verbal consent yet the judge orders you to testify, you have two options. The first is to state for the record your ethical responsibilities to obtain consent. If the judge still orders you to testify, you can provide such testimony or you can refuse. Such refusal may result in your being held in contempt of court or being subjected to other sanctions. Although there are some instances in which defying a court order may be appropriate, it is normally wiser to obey the court after appropriately informing the court about your ethical responsibilities and how complying with the court's request necessarily places you in violation of those responsibilities.

How does a clinician handle confidential information that comes her way even though she has not asked for it? Consider an example where Evelyn has completed her court testimony as an expert witness. The court has made a decision about Debra's custody and visitation, but now Philip has gone back to court for an increase in visitation periods. Philip's lawyer, Lori, asks Freida to release her updated treatment information to Evelyn. For the sake of argument, let us say that Paula agrees to sign the release of information. Should Freida release her treatment information to Evelyn, the court's witness? Freida probably has no ethical issue, since she is responding to a request to release of records by both clients, Philip and Paula. However, what should Evelyn do? Here, again, we have an interesting ethical dilemma. Evelyn no longer is collecting data. Yet, she receives data. Evelyn no longer is formulating her opinion for the court. She has completed her task, having already testified.

Those of us involved in custody evaluations know that high-conflict parents often relitigate. It is not unusual for a court to order an updated evaluation. Evelyn should probably do two things. The first is to file the information without reading it. The second is to write to the judge, with a copy to each attorney, asking for the court's guidance. In some jurisdictions Evelyn may need to write to the attorneys, with a copy to the judge. However, Evelyn probably should do nothing more than file the information until she receives clear directions from the court–not the attorneys. This is an important point. Evelyn is working for the court in her role as its expert. The instruction to perform further work must come from Evelyn's client, the court, not the attorneys. Although they may place a motion before the court requesting that Evelyn assess the new information, it is the court that should direct Evelyn's activities.

Freedom of Information and Privacy Legislation

Some jurisdictions have freedom of information and protection of privacy legislation (at the federal level, see the Freedom of Information Act, 5 USC 552).[14] These laws regulate access to records held by government agencies and some organizations that receive government funding. Whether an organization is covered depends on its contractual relationship with the government. The legislation tries to balance the interests of an individual's privacy, state security, the public's right to know, and freedom of expression.

Privacy legislation (such as the federal Family Educational Rights and Privacy Act of 1994, 20 USC) guarantees protection of privacy for certain types of information. Agencies where the legislation provides specific privacy protection include schools, substance abuse treatment programs, public social services, venereal disease clinics, and other publicly funded medical service providers (Saltzman & Furman, 1999). Professionals who work in these areas cannot release information without explicit written consent of the person who is the subject of the records or upon an order of the court.

The process for applying for information under freedom of information laws is an administrative process with regional differences, so

---

[14]For more information about federal Freedom of Information laws and procedures, see http://www.usdoj.gov/foia/04_3.html.

we will not describe the process in detail. Legislation and regulations explain who to contact for access to information, how to apply, and the criteria for granting and denying access (most states have web sites that include the most recent legislation and guidelines). Agency policies should reflect these laws so that requests can be processed fairly and efficiently.

The fact that a client has obtained information under freedom of information laws does not necessarily make you compellable as a witness. Freedom of information and compellability are treated as separate issues.

Compelling a Clinician to Disclose

When an attorney approaches a clinician to provide information for legal proceedings, the attorney will generally prefer to enlist the clinician on a voluntary basis. Because of the clinician's professional obligations to his clients, he may not be able to disclose information without the client's written consent to release the information. Accordingly, if an attorney takes steps to legally compel you to disclose information, you may wish to challenge the "motion to compel." Remember, just because you have been subpoenaed does not mean that you need to provide what is requested by the subpoena. You are legally required to respond to a subpoena. One appropriate response is to file a "motion to quash." In it, you may explain to the court why protection of your client's confidential information is critical to maintaining the integrity of the therapeutic relationship. It might be useful to present an argument about why the need to protect the information is more important than the need to disclose the information. The legal system often examines the relative merits or weights of conflicting arguments. If you can make a strong case about the harm or detriment caused by the disclosure, such an argument might outweigh the value of disclosing the information, at least disclosing the information in the manner requested by the attorney asking for the information.

If the court agrees with your argument, then you may not have to disclose any information. If the court orders you to provide the requested information, you may have a responsibility to explain to the court the ethical obligation to maintain the confidentiality of the communication and then provide the court with the information requested. You may have an ethical obligation to state for the record how the court's instruction is contrary to your professional ethics. There are times when you may feel strongly about an issue and decide to disobey the order of the court for moral reasons. In doing so, you would put yourself at peril, legally and ethically. Legally, if you are in contempt of court, you could be fined or imprisoned. Ethically, you could face discipline or expulsion from your professional regulatory organization.

Before you respond to any request to provide information to an attorney or the court, stop and think about how disclosure of this information may fit into the larger picture. In some cases you may be relieved to receive a court order because that may take the burden off you to decide whether to disclose. For example, Michael could have had concerns about Freida's methods of practice, but the Carveys may not have provided permission to release any information about such concerns. No matter how strong Michael's feelings may be about the importance of reporting Freida to a licensing board or professional association, if the client holds the privilege of the communication and decides not to provide permission to release such information, Michael has no choice but to respect the wishes of the client.

On the other hand, if Michael were compelled by an order of the court to disclose information about Freida's practices, then he would be allowed to talk about his concerns in a context that encourages scrutiny and responsibility.

Some clinicians may feel unsettled about being compelled by court order to release information. They may feel anxious about testifying. They may feel concerned about their own work coming under attack as a means of diverting the court's attention away from the concerns about Freida's work. They may feel uneasy about having to provide information about a client and the potential effects such disclosure may have on the therapeutic relationship.

There are a variety of ways a clinician can be required to provide testimony or to disclose records. These include police warrants, subpoenas and applications for production, discovery, disclosure, or orders from the court. You should obtain legal advice if you plan to challenge any of these processes. Different tribunals have different degrees of authority to compel witnesses. Typically criminal courts have the greatest authority. Some tribunals have no authority to compel witnesses.

Warrants

A search warrant is a court order permitting police to search a particular location or property to investigate a crime. The police may gather evidence for use in subsequent criminal proceedings. In order to receive a warrant, police must show probable cause that a crime has been committed. The court will try to restrict the scope of the search in order to limit infringement on civil rights. Warrants are generally not used to gain access to a client's records.[15] If you as a clinician are not a suspect in an investigation, you are less likely to be presented with a search warrant than to receive a subpoena or an application for discovery.

Subpoenas

A subpoena[16] is a summons requiring you (the recipient of the subpoena) to appear before a court or other hearing at a particular date, time, and place to give testimony for a particular case. A subpoena may also require you to bring relevant records and documents to a hearing. You may not have to testify or disclose your records upon receipt of a subpoena, but you do have to respond through either compliance or a legal challenge. Consult with your attorney to help you decide whether to provide the information required by the subpoena or to respond with a motion to quash, a request for an *in camera* review, or some other remedy. Refusal to comply with a subpoena is considered contempt of court, with possible punishments including fines or incarceration.

To illustrate, consider a situation where Paula refuses to provide a consent to release confidential information to Freida. Lori subpoenas Freida's treatment notes and assessment information. Freida realizes that failure to respond to the subpoena may result in charges of contempt of court and penalties. On the other hand, Freida has an ethical responsibility to keep Paula's information confidential. So, how can Freida respond to this dilemma?

Let us say that Freida has filed a motion to quash and the judge determines Freida needs to turn over the information to Lori in spite of

---

[15]Police are most likely to use warrants to search an accused person's case files if the person is currently incarcerated or has been incarcerated.

[16]The term "subpoena" is generally used in criminal hearings; other types of proceedings may be empowered to issue a "notice to attend" or similar instrument. For the sake of simplicity, the term subpoena is used throughout this volume.

Paula's continued refusal to release Freida to do so. Although she must respond to the court's order to release the information, Freida also has a responsibility to provide an explanation of her professional ethics and responsibility that is read into the formal record of the trial. In this statement to the court, Freida notes, "I have informed the court of my ethical responsibility to maintain the confidentiality of my professional communications with Freida. Confidentiality is a cornerstone of my practice, as it offers clients a safe and trusting environment to discuss difficult personal issues. Given my professional ethics, I do not agree with the court's decisions, though I will reluctantly comply with the court's order."

If you are served with a subpoena, you may not have to turn over your files nor speak with the attorneys for either party prior to your attendance at the hearing. However, *depending upon your role*, you may decide to meet with a "friendly attorney" or to share information prior to the hearing. Cooperating with an attorney may facilitate settlement and help both you and the attorney prepare for the hearing. If someone other than your client's attorney issues the subpoena, you should inform your client that you have received a subpoena. You may also need to contact your client's attorney upon proper consent. The attorney and you may discuss what steps you plan to take.

If your client does not have an attorney and you receive a subpoena for her records, you should advise the client to obtain independent legal advice. If your client intends to claim privilege, be careful about providing information to the attorneys in advance of the hearing. If you provide information to the attorney for one party, that attorney may have to disclose the information to the attorney for the other party.

There are three potential advantages to being subpoenaed. Since you are being required by the court to testify, you may be viewed as a more objective witness than if you were to cooperate voluntarily with one side. Further, being subpoenaed protects you from a client's claim that you have breached confidentiality when you testify. Third, the subpoena should specify that you are being asked to testify as an expert, which in most states, is tied into statutory requirements that fees be provided for expert witness testimony. If you are subpoenaed by one side, it is that side's responsibility to pay your fees. If you are subpoenaed by the court, it may be the responsibility of the court (or in some states, it may be the responsibility of the administrative office of the court) to pay your fees.

A party can bring a motion to quash the subpoena on the grounds that the information is privileged or the file is irrelevant. Alternatively, a client may claim privilege at the hearing to prevent a clinician from being compelled to testify. The judge has the power to decide on a case-by-case basis whether certain information should be protected by privilege. The decision is made on several bases. One factor is whether the information is needed to determine the case, as balanced against the interests of protecting the confidentiality of the professional relationship. Factors that weigh in favor of making the information available to the court include the seriousness of the issues (e.g., a criminal case with charges of murder) and the lack of other sources of evidence. Factors that weigh in favor of excluding the evidence include the following: people should be encouraged to make use of certain professionals; confidentiality is required to maintain the relationship; the community values this type of relationship; and the harms caused by disclosure are greater than the related benefits. This last factor is often the primary issue to be determined.

Another basis is whether the information to be presented provides information that is more probative than prejudicial. That is, is the information to be presented to the court important to the factual basis of the case, or is it more likely to elicit an emotional response from those who would hear it (such as jurors) that might color the way they view the client?

Consider a case in which Philip is charged with physical assault against Paula. If Philip had been going to a clinician for "anger management," the clinician might have information that could help the prosecution prove that Philip committed the alleged offense. In spite of this benefit, a court might be hesitant about compelling the clinician to testify. Such a disclosure would surely discourage Philip (and others like him) from seeking therapeutic help for anger and violent behavior. Since other sources of evidence are available, including Paula's testimony and physical evidence of assault, the harm caused by forcing disclosure is greater than its benefits.

Even when a clinician is compelled to disclose information, there are ways to limit the harm from disclosure. For example, the attorneys could meet with the judge in her chambers to decide whether particular information should be disclosed and, if so, how. The judge could restrict the scope of the questioning to topics that are most relevant and least disturbing. Further, she could limit who is present at the hearing or prohibit publication by newspapers, television, and other media. These decisions are based on a balancing of the client's right to privacy, the public's right to know, and the accused's right to a fair trial. As noted above, this area of law is full of controversy and in a state of flux, so obtaining legal advice would be wise, should you or your client have questions about a particular case.

Other Applications for Disclosure, Production, or Discovery

After a legal proceeding has been initiated, a party may bring forward other types of applications to compel a clinician to disclose confidential information. Applications for disclosure, production of documents, or discovery are intended to enable each party to have access to information that may most affect its case.[17] Further, a defendant in a case is entitled to know the case that may be brought against her, so that there are no surprises at the hearing. These pretrial disclosure processes may make it easier for the parties to settle the case before trial. (Disclosure processes are discussed further in Chapter 10.)

In criminal proceedings an accused party initiates a disclosure application by serving the clinician or her agency with the application. It will state what records are being requested and the reasons for the request.[18] The client and the prosecution should also receive notice, so that they can speak to the issue. A judge will hear the application. Although you are not required to attend the hearing to determine disclosure, you need to decide whether to appear in court and whether to have an attorney represent you. You may have concerns about the impact of disclosure on your client (e.g., stress, embarrassment, loss of trust). You may also have independent concerns (e.g., whether the records identify other clients, such as family or group members; your ability to produce the documents; whether the records will be used to impugn your reputation). In some cases, professional associations and victim advocate groups have asked for standing to present arguments in such hearings or have helped to pay for a clinician's attorney.

The court will deal with arguments about the relevance of the doc-

---

[17]Note that in criminal cases, only the defense can request and receive disclosure. The defense does not need to reveal its case to the prosecution, except in rare cases.

[18]In most cases, the prosecution just hands over copies of all of its documents. This makes it unnecessary for an application for disclosure to go before a judge.

uments and claims for privilege. The judge may privately review the documents as part of her decision-making process. If the judge determines certain records should not be disclosed, they may still be kept in a sealed envelope and retained by the court until all court proceedings are exhausted. Retaining the documents allows the court to access them if issues are raised during trial that require disclosure. Find out in advance whether the court wants your original records or whether copies are acceptable. If the court requests originals, be sure to keep copies for yourself.

When a criminal court considers an application for disclosure, it must balance the client's right to privacy and the accused's right to a fair trial. The defense must establish that information contained in the records is "likely to be relevant" to the legal issues in the case and "material to the defense." Courts have said they will discourage fishing expeditions as well as obstructive and time-consuming requests for information. This is a particular concern where the defense is harassing a victim-witness.

When assessing whether clinical records must be produced, a court may consider the following factors:

- The extent to which the record is necessary for the accused to make a full answer and defense.
- The probative value of the record (i.e., the soundness of the information as evidentiary proof).
- Whether a client could reasonably expect the record to remain private.
- Whether production of the record would be premised upon any discriminatory belief or bias.
- Potential prejudice to the complainant's dignity, privacy, or security of the person that would be occasioned by production of the record (*Regina v. O'Conner*, 1995).
- The terms of any statutory provisions that provide for confidentiality or privilege of information in specific contexts such as drug and alcohol programs, mental health settings, and schools (Dickson, 1995).

To minimize intrusion into privacy if a court orders records to be produced, the judge may edit what may be disclosed, limit who may have copies, and specify how copies will be returned to their original custodian when court proceedings are completed.[19] If pretrial production is ordered, this information will probably be admissible in court during trial; however, admissibility may be challenged again during trial.

CONCLUSION

You do not want to be caught off guard when an attorney or client initially raises a concern that has legal implications. Basically you need to consider four questions:

1. What are my legal and professional obligations in terms of client confidentiality, privilege, and protection of individuals from harm to themselves or others?
2. How do I respond to a complaint in a manner that is most likely to satisfy the complainant's concerns without putting myself or others at risk (psychologically, physically, legally, or financially)?
3. When information about a client is requested, should I provide the information voluntarily or refuse until I am requested to do so by law (e.g., through a subpoena or court order)?
4. Should I contact my attorney, superior, colleague, insurer, or professional association for advice and support?

Watch for red flags in your everyday practice that suggest that you should seek legal consultation. In some situations the need for legal advice is quite obvious: being served with a claim, subpoena, or other legal document; assessing a client's risk of committing suicide or homicide; being confronted by a client who is hostile or otherwise demonstrates a proclivity to litigation; and identifying a situation where you may have caused emotional, physical, or financial damage to a client. Other situations will require your best judgment call—for example, a

---

[19]Bring copies and your original records to the hearing. If you are prepared to testify that the copy is an exact (true) one, then the judge may allow you to keep the originals and provide copies to the other parties.

father coming into treatment to talk about what children need when living with only one parent, or a mother refusing to allow you to read relevant documents on advice of her attorney. Err on the safe side.

Ideally you will have a trusted attorney on retainer who is readily accessible for consultation. In addition, your practice will have established policies that provide guidelines for confidentiality and how to respond to various legal contingencies.

Chapter 4

Preparation for Legal Proceedings

Assume that you have agreed to cooperate with a "friendly attorney" who has contacted you as a potential witness and that you have dealt with any concerns about confidentiality. In some situations, the attorney will inform you about the time and location of the hearing, but provide little other information. If your role as a witness is relatively minor and straightforward, this may be sufficient. For example, Michael may be called to testify about his knowledge that Philip and Paula attended mediation. If the rest of Michael's information is deemed privileged, meeting with the attorney in advance may be unnecessary. If you are called as a witness and believe that a meeting with an attorney would be useful, do not hesitate to ask for one. There is always a balancing act required. In this case, the balancing act is between the need to consult with the attorney and the costs of such a meeting to your client. Remember that the attorney is being paid by her client for time spent on the case. So, if you ask for a meeting, it will cost your client money. Consider ways to avoid running up costs: communicate in writing or by telephone rather than in person, keep discussions focused and minimize travel when you do meet in person.[1] Attorneys often prefer meetings at their own offices.

---

[1] Some law firms try to contain legal costs by employing junior attorneys for the preparation phase. A junior attorney may have more time to spend and provide competent services. If you are working with a junior attorney and have any concerns, raise them with the junior attorney first, but do not hesitate to contact the attorney who is ultimately responsible for the case, if need be.

Before meeting with the attorney, review your case notes and ensure that they are in order. "Tampering" with notes may be considered an obstruction of justice, so do not make changes to original documents, including whiting out, deleting, or destroying them. Missing pages and different writing styles are easy tipoffs to tampering. If you need to make corrections or additions, then write your new notes in a way that clearly shows they were added after the fact. State your reasons for the corrections or additions and include the date when you recorded them. These steps will show that you are not trying to cover up something. Prepare an executive summary for yourself as a way to focus your thoughts and describe the order of events. Bring notes, documentation, and questions that you want to discuss with the attorney.

When you arrange for a meeting, ask the attorney about her purposes for the meeting. Typically, if an attorney wants to meet with you at this stage, it is to gather information to build her case, to test your credibility, and to determine whether to call you as a witness. Your information may facilitate a negotiated agreement or be used at a trial of the issues. It is often useful to ask the attorney to define a set of questions that she wants you to address. This would allow you to consider your answers prior to meeting with the attorney.

In this chapter we describe the processes of gathering information and the decision about whether to call a clinician as a witness. In the latter part of this chapter we elaborate on how a clinician can prepare for a particular legal proceeding once he knows he is going to be called as a witness.

GATHERING INFORMATION[2]

When gathering information, the attorney wants to know as much about the case as possible. Accordingly, she will ask for information that is both favorable and unfavorable to her client's case. Both you and the attorney have a mutual interest in finding out "what really happened," although either of you may have a propensity to color the truth in favor of your client. When you meet with the attorney, be clear and deliberate about the role you are playing—are you an advocate for your client, a

---

[2]This section describes an in-depth process of gathering information. In many cases, due to time, cost, and other practical considerations, this process is abridged.

fact witness, or an expert witness? Even when acting as an advocate, if you were to lie or withhold certain information, you would likely be acting unethically or illegally.[3] And such actions may come back to haunt you in later proceedings.

To facilitate information gathering, the attorney will ideally engage you in a way that enables you to open up and recall events as accurately as possible. An effective interviewer will begin by asking general questions, followed by closed or focused questions to elicit more detail. Accordingly, the beginning of the interview will provide the best opportunity to give an overview of information you think is relevant. Because focused questions may sometimes lead to a distorted view, try to remember the facts as accurately as possible and avoid the temptation of telling the attorney exactly what you think she most wants to hear. It is much better to confront the attorney with adverse or qualified information at this stage than to allow surprises to arise at later stages of the proceedings.

As the attorney asks more focused questions, you may become aware of the issues that are important from a legal perspective—what evidence is needed to defend against fraud, discrimination, deportation, negligence, breach of contract, or whatever issue is at stake. An attorney builds his case by identifying the relevant legal issues and the evidence required to establish the allegations or defense. The parties may agree on some facts. If the case goes to a hearing, each side only has to prove the facts in dispute. If the information you provide is solid or indisputable, you may not have to be called as a witness since both parties will likely accept your information as fact. This is called a stipulation. The parties may stipulate to your information coming in as evidence without asking for your testimony.

The attorney may try to obtain your version of what happened by taking you through a historical reconstruction of events in chronological order. Since most adjudications focus on what happened in the past, the attorney will want to know what information you have concerning critical incidents.

This area of inquiry may hold significant areas of concern for you. Typically, your testimony is about what a client has reported to you

---

[3]Some would say lying or withholding information is always unethical. However, others would say there are some rare exceptions where a value higher than honesty can ethically justify dishonesty (e.g., to save a life) (Loewenberg et al., 2000).

about an event that has occurred outside of the therapy office. Your so-called version of what happened, in fact, is your interpretation and reci-tation of what you have been told by the client about what happened. It is likely not a direct observation of the alleged event in question. Do not get caught up in trying to argue for the truth of your client's version as repeated to you during therapy. Your knowledge is limited to what the client reported about an event. Your knowledge is about the client's rep-resentation of a specific event rather than about your independent im-pressions about the event unless you were present to witness the event itself.

There is case law in the United States that reminds us that mental health professionals are not in the role of judging the credibility of wit-nesses, and in this particular context your client may be a witness (*State of Oregon v. Milbrandt*, 1988). The role of determining the credibility of a witness is left to the trier of fact, either the judge or the jury. The clini-cian's role is to provide information that may be helpful to the trier of fact. If you are admitted as a fact witness, your role is to provide factual information. Technically, a fact witness may provide no opinions. Therefore, if you are asked to testify as a fact witness, you may be un-able to play the role of advocate. Since an advocate holds an opinion about the rightness of a particular perspective, the role of an advocate is to provide an opinion about what you believe to be right. It is therefore not within the province of a fact witness to testify in an advocacy role.[4]

Although some attorneys are quite formal when they interview witnesses, this process is much different than being examined or cross-examined at a hearing. The range of information that you discuss with the attorney will be much broader than what would be permissible in a hearing. In private discussions with the attorney you are generally freer to reflect without as much concern for being clear, concise, and com-pletely consistent. The attorney will use these early discussions to de-termine which information is relevant, admissible, and necessary to be presented if the case proceeds to a hearing.

To help you better recall the therapy sessions, the attorney may ask you to review exhibits filed in court or go back through your notes. Such requests may be annoying if you believe that you have already re-

---

[4]For further information about the definition and testimonial limitations of fact and expert witnesses, consult either the Federal Rules of Evidence or your state's evidence code.

lated everything you know. However, if you comply with such suggestions, you may well be surprised at what else you remember.

The safest bet is to rely on your notes and memory. Although use of techniques such as visualization and other recall aids may be useful during a discussion with an attorney outside of court, the usefulness of information recalled during such exercises is highly suspect. Although most clinicians are aware of the highly suggestible nature of memory recollection in young children (Ceci & Bruck, 1995; Faller & Scarenecchia, 1998; Poole & Lamb, 1998), there also is considerable research indicating similar suggestibility for adult memories, as well (Loftus & Ketcham, 1991). Thus, providing testimony about information that was retrieved using a memory aid such as visualization may leave you open to attacks on the reliability of the information as well as on your credibility as a professional who appears unaware of relevant research pertaining to information retrieval and recall. Our advice: stick to what you know and what is in your notes.

You may be asked to relate specific incidents and examples by breaking up large events into smaller components. The seemingly mundane detail requested by attorneys may frustrate you. Remember the level of detail a witness can provide is used as evidence that the witness recalls an event accurately. If an attorney focuses on discrete events, you may feel she is losing sight of the big picture. Although the attorney will have reasons for her line of questions, this is a time when you can raise your concerns about the broader picture. For example, Lori may ask Freida questions about isolated incidents in which Paula made threats toward Philip. Freida may need to help Lori to consider the broader context of these outbursts: Paula's reaction to separation, fears that her daughter would be abducted, and her limited knowledge of her legal rights.

It is important to remember that, when people do not recall details of events, they often fill in the blanks with information that makes sense either from the perspective of today's recall or based upon knowledge of situations that are similar to those of the particular event. Unless you have a clear memory represented in written notes, you are on somewhat shaky ground in providing such testimony. We know from memory research that human beings tend to fill in blanks with information drawn from their experience in similar situations. We also know that such memory completion tasks may make one feel as though one is accurately representing the past event—and yet be highly inaccurate.

For example, drawing upon the memory research on mothers and children, we know that when asked to immediately recall what their young children's verbatim statements were about an exchange, mothers were notoriously inaccurate in recalling the statements verbatim. They were very good at recalling the general meaning of the statement—called gist memory—but they were very poor at recalling the specific words accurately (Bruck, Ceci, & Francoeur, 1999).

The conclusion is that taking contemporaneous notes during a session and providing only the information drawn from those sessions during testimony best serve clinicians.[5] The further away from the event, the more likely that the memory of the event has been affected by other experiences. It is difficult to testify about your memory of an historical event, given that your memory may be clouded by months or years of intervening therapy with the client as well as therapy with other clients. Be prepared for an attorney to challenge your memory as well as your professional awareness of memory functioning, suggestibility, and recording keeping.

The attorney may ask about practices and events that are of such a normal course that you do not even remember doing them. As a common practice, for example, you as a therapist may routinely screen for suicidal and homicidal ideation. Nonetheless, your notes may not indicate you did a screening unless during the session there was an indication of a crisis. In such circumstances, information on general practices will be useful for the attorney if she wants to establish that the client was not homicidal.

This is a critical point to scrutinize. If your testimony includes that you followed your usual and customary procedures during a treatment session (including screening for suicidal and homicidal ideation), then your written notes would need to reflect this. If you do not have a written record of such inquiry, be careful that your testimony differentiates between your general practice and the specific practice behaviors reflected in your notes for this particular case.

Try to separate out what you know firsthand from what you know from other sources. This may direct the attorney to other sources of evidence, including witnesses, records, or documents. If you are reluctant

---

[5]Recent research indicates that even verbatim contemporaneous notes are susceptible to numerous mistakes when matched against audiotaped records of those same interview sessions (Lamb, Orbach, Sternberg, Hershkowitz, & Horowitz, 2000).

to testify, identifying other sources may provide an opportunity for the attorney to find a more willing witness. It may be a good idea to talk with these potential witnesses first about their willingness to testify before you provide the attorney with their names and phone numbers. It is a professional courtesy to inform a colleague.

To facilitate information gathering, it is helpful if the attorney is familiar with scientific knowledge from your field of clinical practice. Sam, for example, can help to educate the attorney for his child protection agency about current research findings about the physical and psychological attributes most closely associated with child maltreatment. It might also be important to provide the attorney with rival but plausible alternative perspectives that undercut or contradict the current conventional wisdom. In this way the attorney can be made more knowledgeable about the strengths and weaknesses of current research as well as possible professional controversy that may surround the research (e.g., prediction of dangerousness). This incremental knowledge will enable the attorney to ask more informed questions. Conversely, the greater your own familiarity with the law, the better you will be at providing information that is significant from the attorney's perspective. Familiarity with one another's jargon will help you avoid miscommunication, particularly when legal definitions of terms differ from psychological or sociological meanings. Although you may feel knowledgeable about the law, be careful about wresting control of the information-gathering process from the attorney. Telling a lawyer how to do her job may be analogous to a client who comes to you with a little knowledge about psychology and then tries to tell you how to conduct psychotherapy with him.

Ask the attorney for information about relevant case law, statutes, and local rules that are relevant to your testimony.[6] Also, ask about what *not* to say on the stand. In some personal injury cases, for example, an attorney might advise an expert not to testify about his conclusions, as these might adversely affect the size of the monetary award.

Remember to ask questions about how attorneys use words that may appear familiar to us as mental health professionals. For example, in legal parlance the term "reliable" is used in a manner somewhat akin

---

[6]See "Websites for Legal Research" in the References section for a list of websites to aid clinicians in accessing this information themselves. Although you may be able to do some of your own legal research to gain a general understanding of the law, specific legal research requires training to ensure you are accessing the most current, relevant laws.

to statistician's use of the term "valid." Asking for definitions as needed will help clarify what specific information you are being asked to discuss. Do not assume that just because you are both repeating the same words that you are necessarily speaking the same language or communicating the same thoughts!

SENSITIVE INFORMATION

Even in situations where you have a client's permission to discuss confidential information with the attorney, be cautious about *how* you share sensitive information and set conditions, as needed, on how that information might be used. For example, if you share information about your client with her attorney, can that information be shared with the client? Is there an ethical obligation to disclose such information to your client before you talk with the attorney? Sam could be concerned about Paula's safety. He could ask the attorney not to tell Philip where Paula is staying. If you need to establish terms of confidentiality for the sake of the client's safety or mental welfare, negotiate, and document these terms before disclosing sensitive information.

In a variation, if you share opinions rather than simply facts with the attorney, do you have a responsibility to share those same opinions with your client? Do you have an obligation to discuss those opinions with your client *before* talking with the attorney? In determining how to approach these questions, be clear about your primary responsibility. As a clinician, your primary responsibility is to your client. Therefore, any opinions expressed to your client's attorney need to be discussed first with your client, both as a matter of ethics as well as a matter of good sense. By reviewing with your client all that you expect to say to her attorney, you define the limits of what you will discuss and provide an opportunity to work with your client on how such information is to be presented to someone outside of the treatment session. This type of review provides the client with a greater sense of safety and trust.

Conversely, an attorney may be unable to tell you everything about a case due to attorney–client privilege or for strategic reasons. The attorney may have investigated you before the interview to explore your knowledge and motivation. She may not want to tell you too much in order to hear your evidence freshly and to avoid biasing you. Another reason an attorney may not share information or strategy with you is to avoid placing you in a situation in which you would have to testify about what you know about aspects of the case that are unrelated to your client's condition but perhaps relevant to the overall legal position. If you find the attorney is withholding important information from you, inquire about the reasons for doing so.

THE DECISION TO CALL YOU AS A WITNESS

During the information-gathering process, the attorney will assess whether to call you as a witness. At this point, there is no ownership of witnesses. If the attorney who initially interviews you decides not to call you as a witness, the attorney for the other party may still call you. Whether you respond to the second attorney's call depends upon the nature of the relationship between you and the first attorney. If you have been hired by the first attorney, any communication acknowledging your involvement may be privileged. If you have not been hired by the first attorney, you may be free to talk with the second attorney.

Two questions will determine whether you will be called as a witness: Do you have useful evidence, and will you make an effective witness? In terms of the first question, the attorney will consider whether you have any observations that are vital to proving his case. (The attorney may also want you to present opinion evidence, as described in Chapter 7 on expert witnesses.) The attorney will have to decide if any other sources can provide the same information as you and compare how strong each source is. For example, if the choice is between a live witness and written information, the attorney may decide to enter the documents as evidence, because the attorney can never be sure what a witness will say on the stand. More than one source of information may be needed to prove certain facts, so you could be called to attest to the information in a document or to corroborate the testimony of another witness. Although some hearings go on for months or years, most hearings are short-lived, most typically taking hours rather than days. There are also pressures to keep costs down, which may limit the number of witnesses to be called. The attorney must also consider whether the tribunal will make certain inferences if a particular witness is not called to testify.

As noted in Chapter 2, an effective witness is one who is *credible*. To assess your credibility, the attorney may ask questions concerning the following:

- *Motivation*: How cooperative will you be as a witness? How objective are your information and beliefs? Do you have an interest in the outcome of the case? Will you be perceived as having biases toward one party or the other? How do you define your therapeutic role (e.g., supportive, confronting)?
- *Perception*: How accurate is your perception of what happened (e.g., accuracy of sight, hearing, interpretation of stimuli)? What were the effects of environmental and circumstantial factors affecting perception (e.g., lighting, noise, fatigue, stress, biases from the clinician's theoretical perspective)? Did you observe the information directly, or is it secondhand information?
- *Memory*: How accurate is your recall? How certain are you about your facts?
- *Communication skills*: How well can you articulate your recollections? Are you able to focus on the facts? How well do you communicate under pressure?

In order to ascertain your credibility, the attorney will not ask these questions directly, but will look for subtle indicators: Do you tend to agree with the questioner? Is your story consistent? Do you have past experiences that may color your perceptions? How have you testified in previous cases? While your interview with the attorney in private is not a cross-examination, questions about your credibility may help prepare you for cross-examination at a hearing. She may ask you, for example, "How do you remember this client so clearly?" Try to be direct and honest with the attorney. Consider an information-gathering meeting between Lori and Freida. Freida might become defensive if Lori asked about her methods of assessment. If Freida can be open about the deficiencies in her assessment, Lori can help with how to confront them to minimize embarrassment when Freida is testifying. If Freida discloses her biases, Lori and Freida can deal with these, possibly deciding to find a less biased clinician to testify instead of Freida.

The attorney may be blunt with you concerning whether you will be a useful witness. You may find this uncomfortable. In most legal processes, attorneys decide who will be called as a witness. If you believe that you should be called, but the attorneys indicate that you will not, secure legal advice to determine whether there is a means for you to participate in the hearing (e.g., by preparing an *amicus curiae*, or friend-of-the-court brief).

On the other hand, you may be reluctant to testify. If you want to dissuade the attorney from calling you as a witness, you could exhibit poor memory, poor clinical skills, or evidence contrary to the attorney's case. If any of these portrayals is fictitious, consider the potential consequences.[7] Even leaving aside the ethical questions and professional obligations, consider whether you will really achieve what you intend. For example, a sexual abuse counselor might consider "intentionally forgetting" everything that happened in your clinical intervention with a particular client. Does this really advance the client's interests? If the counselor's performance of incompetence is accepted, how will this affect the counselor's reputation in the community and with the professional regulatory association? Are there any alternatives to protect the client's interests? Could the counselor talk to the attorney about his or her reluctance to testify?

Even if an attorney initially decides to call you as a witness, you may not actually have to testify. The case may settle before or even during a hearing. Alternatively, the other party may admit the facts to which you were to testify, negating the need to call you as a witness.

SIGNED STATEMENTS

There are times when an attorney may request that you sign a statement attesting to the information you provided. A signed statement serves several purposes. If the statement is about a recent event, it may be used later to refresh your memory or to support your evidence. Providing a written statement ensures that you focus your thoughts and commit to a specific version of what happened. On the downside, a signed statement may be used to find inconsistencies in your evidence at a subse-

---

[7]Consequences for dishonesty may include being sued by a client or other individual who suffers as a result, being charged with fraud or obstruction of justice, being fired or disciplined by one's employer, and being disciplined by one's professional association. Also consider societal obligations as a citizen to act in a manner that promotes social justice.

quent hearing. The statement could also make you feel that you cannot add to or change your testimony later on. If you do want to make changes, advise the attorney as soon as possible.

Do not feel pressured into signing a statement. Let the attorney know if you need more time to think about what happened or to go over your records. Ask the attorney to prepare a summary of the important facts and give you a copy to review with your agency or attorney. You can then suggest changes and sign the statement only when you feel completely comfortable with the specific language used. If you discover an error in your original statement, it is better to add truthful amendments than to try to appear infallible. As an alternative to a signed statement, you may request to audiotape or videotape your information.

PREPARING FOR A HEARING

Assume that you have been subpoenaed or have agreed to participate as a witness and that you are now ready to prepare for testifying. Some attorneys believe too much preparation can hurt the effectiveness of a witness; a witness who is too polished may not come across as credible, while a witness who knows a good deal about the law may second-guess his attorney's strategies. However, an informed witness has a greater sense of control over the process and the capacity to be a better witness. The potential consequences in legal proceedings are too important to risk learning by "trial and error." As a clinician, you endeavor to be competent as a practitioner. In your role as a witness, there is no less reason to strive for competence. In this section we deal with the following components for competence as a witness: What knowledge do you need, what skills can you practice, and how can you psychologically and emotionally prepare yourself? This section also takes up ethical issues that can arise in the context of preparation.

A variety of factors will affect the amount of preparation you will need for a particular case, including your past experience, familiarity with legal processes and issues, confidence in public speaking, reaction to time pressures, outstanding emotional issues, the importance of the issues to be tried, and whether the proceedings will be televised. Regardless of whether you are involved for the first or thousandth time, do not underestimate the value of preparation.

Knowledge

You could ask the attorney calling you as a witness, "What do I need to know to prepare for the hearing?" The attorney may have standard written or oral information to provide you. If you create your own checklist, you can ask informed questions and assume more responsibility for your preparation. In this section we will discuss the informational aspects of testimony preparation that may assist you, including information about the hearing process, roles of the participants, rules of evidence, substantive law, case facts, and clinical theory.

The Hearing Process

Although you can learn about the hearing process by asking questions or by reading an excellent book on the topic, observing a hearing ahead of time is invaluable preparation. You will gain a feel for the room and the players that can be found only through personal experience. Most court processes are open to the public. Some types of hearings are closed to respect the privacy of participants. If you ask a clerk or administrator responsible for the hearing, you can often gain admittance to observe a closed hearing for the purposes of professional education. Arrange for someone familiar with the process to attend the hearing with you to point out subtleties and answer questions you may have. Make appointments to meet with various participants in the legal process: investigators, district attorneys and their prosecutors, public defenders or legal aid officials, administrative personnel or members of the tribunal. Offer to have lunch *with* them (*buying* them lunch may be construed as a payoff or inappropriate influence). You can use such meetings not only to learn about the process but also to develop a positive rapport with key actors prior to being involved in an actual case with them. You can thereby establish your professionalism, competence, and interest in being a good witness.

At the most basic level, you need to know *where* the hearing will take place, *when* you are expected to be there, and even where you can park your car. Courts generally post dockets, which are daily schedules that you can check for the time and room. Find out from your attorney if you need to let a clerk know that you are present and what your role in the case is (e.g., plaintiff or witness). Your attorney may want you to arrive early, to allow for a final briefing or possibly settlement negotiations. For expediency, some attorneys hold off on meeting with clients or witnesses until just before the hearing. Although you may encourage your attorney to prepare you in advance, you may have to put up with last-minute preparations.

Find out how long you will be expected to wait, the probability of any extended delay, and whether you should wait in the hearing room or outside. Delays can be caused by witnesses not showing up, the testimony of others going overtime, and adjournments for assorted reasons. Bring reading or work that you can do while you wait. Although you may have little choice about when you will be called as a witness, advise the attorney of the times when you absolutely cannot attend and when you are most readily available. An attorney has ethical obligations to inconvenience witnesses as little as possible and to provide sufficient notice for hearings or other processes. Maintain contact with the attorney prior to your testimony in order to keep up with any changes.

For obvious practical reasons, the best time to be scheduled as a witness is the first thing in the morning. Everyone is fresh and able to focus on your evidence. Also, there is less opportunity for something unforeseen to happen and cause delays. For tactical reasons, other concerns may prevail. For example, the opening and closing witnesses are generally assumed to have the greatest impact on the judge and jurors.

Ask if any restrictions prior to giving testimony apply to you. Freida could be asked to stay outside of the hearing room until it is her turn to take the stand. Michael could be asked not to have any further discussions with Philip or Paula. Sam could be sequestered, that is, kept away from the hearing and any other possible sources of information about the case (e.g., media or people involved in the case). The purpose of such restrictions is to ensure that one witness is not influenced by what else is said in or about the hearing. Excluding a witness from the hearing room prior to her testimony is a common procedure. The other restrictions are used sparingly because of their costs and impositions. If a case is likely to attract media attention, ask for advice about how to deal with reporters. Should any reporter actually approach you, a simple "No comment," will normally suffice.

If you are anxious or if this is your first time testifying, consider bringing a support person to sit with while waiting to testify, preferably someone who is calm, reassuring, and sufficiently familiar with the proceedings to answer last-minute questions. If the person is your attorney or an agency colleague, he may also be someone to debrief with afterwards (to review your performance on the stand, give you feedback, and help you with any emotional blows). Some clinicians offer to support their clients by sitting with them during the hearing. Although sitting with a client may be desirable from a clinical standpoint, consider possible implications. If Freida sits with Philip in a custody proceeding, she may appear biased against Paula. Alternatively, Freida may decide to sit with Philip at a circle sentencing process[8] to demonstrate that she supports him. Consider whether escorting your client will distract you from your function as a witness.

Identify what you need to bring to the hearing. In some cases, the attorney will have organized all the documents you need and filed them with the clerk. You should not bring anything to the stand unless you have arranged to do so with the attorney, because anything you bring to the stand could be examined and admitted as evidence. Check whether any of the following should be filed in court, or whether you should bring them: case notes, client records, relevant books or articles, and your *curriculum vitae.*

Roles of Participants

Try to gain a sense of who will be present at the hearing, where everyone will be located, and what their roles will be.[9] In a typical hearing, the judge or person chairing the proceedings will sit at the front of the room, perhaps on an elevated dais. A clerk and a person recording the evidence will sit next to or in front of the dais. The location where you will testify, the witness stand, will be nearby. Ask your attorney if you will be standing or sitting when giving your testimony. In most jurisdictions in the United States, witnesses sit in a witness box. If there is a jury, then the jury box is usually off to one side. There may be separate tables for each party and their attorneys to sit at, located between the judge and the public gallery. As a nonparty witness, you will probably sit in the gallery before you are called to testify. If you are testifying as an expert witness, generally you are allowed to listen to and incorporate

---

[8]This process is an alternative to standard criminal justice proceedings that is used most often in Native American communities.

[9]Knowing the name of each key person may also be useful, since people generally respond more positively when you address them by name (e.g., "Mr. Li," rather than "Sir" or "Counselor"). This also demonstrates that you have a good memory.

trial testimony into your own testimony. As a fact witness, you may be sequestered to prevent your being influenced by other testimony.

Security guards or officers may be present. Certain officials in the room may have hidden call buttons in case there is an emergency. If, as a clinician, you are aware of potentially dangerous behavior by a client, consider advising your attorney to arrange for appropriate precautions.[10]

The judge or equivalent is responsible for chairing the process, ensuring that decorum is maintained, and ruling on any procedural issues. Judges may ask witnesses questions; depending on the type of tribunal and the issues involved, some adjudicators take on a more active and investigative role. If there is no jury, the judge also hears the evidence and legal arguments, makes findings of fact, and renders decisions by applying relevant laws to the facts of the case.

The clerk or registrar assists the adjudicator. A clerk's duties include opening and closing the hearing, ensuring appropriate people are present, carrying out administrative procedures for the hearing, marking exhibits, and swearing in witnesses. The person who records the evidence may be a stenographer, oral recorder, or person who runs audio-recording equipment. The typed or audiotaped recording is used to prepare a verbatim transcript of the proceedings.

Parties are individuals or institutions that have brought the matter to trial (e.g., a plaintiff or an applicant) or are being brought to trial (e.g., a defendant or a respondent). Each party may represent himself or herself. This is called acting *pro se*. In more formal hearings, parties generally use attorneys. In some proceedings a party may use a nonattorney advocate. However, in most court proceedings an advocate must be licensed to practice law.

In her role as an advocate, the attorney is expected to decide the legal theory of the case, what evidence to present and how to present it. She will determine which witnesses to call and the order of the evidence. She will examine the witnesses she calls and cross-examine the witnesses the other party calls. She may object to questions from the

---

[10]We have known clinicians who have received death threats from clients who were angry about the information they expected the clinician to introduce into evidence. If you receive threats from a client, do not hesitate to consult with others, such as your attorney or supervisor or the client's attorney, to help assess the threat and to determine what actions to take. Backing away from giving testimony would not be an appropriate way to resolve the problem.

other party based on rules of evidence. As a witness, you may feel that you have little control over this process. The more familiar you are with the law and the greater the trust you have built with the attorney, the greater your opportunity to work on a more equal basis with the attorney, at least at this preparation stage. For example, Evelyn may have suggestions about what evidence tends to be persuasive with a particular judge, or Sam may be able to suggest questions that Lori can ask him. The attorney and clinician should recognize the strengths and limitations of the other's training and background, as well as the need to differentiate their roles.

The primary role of a witness is to present information under oath or affirmation. Oath refers to swearing or promising to tell the truth, placing one's hand on a Bible or other holy book. If the witness chooses not to swear on a holy book, he may state that he wishes to "affirm" (promise to tell the truth). A person who makes an oath or affirmation acknowledges the legal and moral consequences that may arise if he commits perjury (i.e., intentionally misleads or lies to the court). Let the attorney know of your intention about making an oath or affirmation. Most hearings will have copies of a Christian Bible readily available. If you want to swear on another holy book (such as the Muslim Koran or Jewish Bible), make arrangements with the attorney in advance. It may be easiest to bring your own holy book.

Rules of Evidence

Evidence is information presented at a hearing to prove facts that must be proved before dealing with the legal issues raised by a case (e.g., facts needed to prove refugee status, malpractice, etc.). The basic rule of evidence for witnesses in court[11] is that they may testify only about facts *within their personal knowledge* regarding issues that are *legally relevant* to the case. (Expert witnesses may provide opinion evidence as well as facts; see Chapter 7.) You can skip down to the next section if you want,

---

[11]Depending on the type of proceeding, there are different standards for what information can be admitted. We will focus on court proceedings in this section, as the rules of evidence in this realm are most developed. Even if "questionable" evidence is admissible in other proceedings, information that follows strict rules of evidence will generally have the greatest impact. Criminal proceedings tend to enforce evidentiary rules most strictly. Family court and child protection proceedings tend to be less formal. Administrative and legislative hearings vary greatly but are generally less rigid than criminal hearings about evidence.

because evidentiary decisions are complex and ultimately the responsibility of judges and attorneys anyhow. If you can weed your way through this section, it will help you understand what makes "good evidence" and how you can tailor what you say in order to maximize its impact. While actually on the stand, you do not want to become preoccupied with the rules of evidence.

Evidence can be classified in different ways:

- Testimonial versus documentary versus real.
- Direct versus circumstantial versus hearsay.
- Fact versus opinion.

Testimonial evidence is information presented under oath by a live witness at the hearing. *Documentary evidence* consists of client files, written assessments, affidavits, or other records filed or entered into the proceedings at the hearing (see Chapters 6 and 8). *Real evidence* includes things that "speak for themselves," for example, a person who shows the court she still has scars or bruising, a picture of a house, or a tape recording of a session. Multiple sources of evidence are often used to corroborate the validity of one another. For example, Sam's records show that Philip behaved in a cooperative manner during his assessment. Sam could also testify to this observation.

Direct evidence is information that establishes the proposition without requiring inferences. Consider a case in which the prosecutor wanted to prove that Philip assaulted Debra. If Paula observed him assault Debra, she could provide direct evidence by testifying about what she saw.

Circumstantial evidence requires inferences to prove the proposition. Consider Paula's evidence that Debra had bruises following three weekend visits with her father. Inferences are based on generalizations: children do not generally get bruises only on weekends. Research knowledge can be used to link circumstantial evidence with the propositions trying to be proved: What are the most common causes of bruises for children of Debra's age? Direct evidence is stronger evidence than circumstantial, because contrary inferences can be drawn from circumstantial evidence. A lot of information presented at a hearing is circumstantial. If there were strong direct evidence, then the case would probably be resolved without the need for a full hearing of the issues.

Hearsay evidence is secondhand information offered for the truth of the statement. The person testifying did not directly observe the events being described, and only knows what she has heard from someone who allegedly observed the events. As a general rule, hearsay is inadmissible in court because the person who made the statement is not on the stand and cannot be questioned to check the truth, accuracy, and meaning of the words or their context.

The admissibility of hearsay evidence is particularly confusing because its admissibility often depends on how the information is to be used. Consider a situation where Paula disclosed to Freida that Philip repeatedly hit Debra. Freida might not be allowed to testify about what Paula said in order to prove that Philip abused Debra. Freida *might* be allowed to testify about what was recorded in her notes. That is, Freida might be allowed to testify about the fact of the statement being in her notes but not about the truthfulness or falsity of the statement.

Paula would be a better witness for this purpose because she is the one who says she observed the alleged abuse. However, if there were a defamation suit against Paula, Freida could testify that she heard Paula make that statement in order to prove that Paula made those statements.

Several exceptions to the hearsay rule exist. They are contexts in which the hearsay statements tend to be reliable. For example, an admission by the accused tends to be reliable because the accused would have no incentive to lie about something that goes against her own interests. Consider a situation in which Philip told Sam, "I hit Debra with a shoe when she wouldn't eat dinner." Sam would be permitted to testify about Philip's admission. On the other hand, Sam might not be allowed to testify that Debra's teacher told him that Philip hit his daughter. Another hearsay exception that has particular relevance to clinicians concerns business records. Records made in the "ordinary course" of clinical work by clinicians at or near the time of contact with the client are admissible even if they contain hearsay. Because the records were kept out of routine rather than in contemplation of a legal action, the contents of the records are likely to be reliable. Other hearsay exceptions are made out of necessity in that there may be no other way to prove certain facts.

Many tribunals have recognized that putting children on the stand to testify is not in the child's best interest. In some cases a clinician will be permitted to interview the child and present the child's statements in the hearing on behalf of the child, notwithstanding the general rule against hearsay. An informal exception to the hearsay rule occurs when a tribunal admits hearsay evidence related to the facts that are uncontested or unimportant to the ultimate decisions to be made. Often, for the sake of convenience, it is easier to permit hearsay rather than to call additional witnesses and require strict proof of every fact.

When you are a witness, try to focus on direct evidence. If the only way you can answer a certain question is by hearsay evidence, you may say that you have no direct knowledge. On the other hand, you could provide your hearsay evidence. If the evidence is ruled inadmissible, do not take it personally. You provided the best information you had. Some attorneys will strategically ask questions that they know will lead to an inadmissible response. Even if the answer is ruled inadmissible, the impact of the response may already have achieved its purpose. After all, it is hard for an adjudicator to completely forget—or rule out of mind—what he has just heard.

Fact evidence is information that is attested to from firsthand observation, perception, or experience. For example, Evelyn could testify about what she heard, saw, felt, smelled, tasted, and did when she conducted a home visit.

Opinion evidence includes beliefs, thoughts, or recommendations that go beyond simple facts. Based on the home visit, did Evelyn express an opinion that Debra's psychological best interests were best served by a residential placement with her mother? Only "expert witnesses" are permitted to provide such opinions (see Chapter 7). Other witnesses are limited to testifying about facts, enabling the judge to draw her own inferences, conclusions, and recommendations.

The best evidence is direct, credible, and original. If a fact can be proven in more than one way, then the attorney should lead with the best evidence (e.g., an original document rather than a photocopy or evidence from a direct witness rather than hearsay). Evidence that is admissible may be afforded different weight by the adjudicator. As a witness, you will want to present information in a way that is not just admissible but also persuasive.[12]

The legal standards for what is relevant in the case may be quite

---

[12]You might wish to consult the Specialty Guidelines for Forensic Psychologists (CEGFP, 1991), which address the appropriateness of advocating for positions supported by the relevant data.

different from what you as a clinician think is relevant.[13] That is, what is legally relevant may be different from what is psychologically relevant. Consider the story of a man who stole a loaf of bread to feed his family. A clinician may believe that the man should not be found criminally responsible due to extenuating circumstances. Lady Justice, however, wears a blindfold to signify that justice is blind. Accordingly, whether the man was hungry when he stole the bread has no legal relevance to the question of whether he committed the crime.[14] During the initial hearing, his clinician would not be allowed to offer testimony about his family circumstances. In criminal trials character testimony is usually not admissible. However, if the defendant is found guilty, the law does permit testimony about character to be admitted into evidence through testimony. Such potentially mitigating evidence may be brought forward in the clinician's presentence report or in direct testimony. While the clinician may find such distinctions artificial and unfair, they are of great importance from a legal perspective. To determine what evidence is relevant, you need to know the legal issues in dispute as well as become familiar with your state's civil and criminal evidence code.

Substantive Law

To be an effective witness, a clinician does not need to be familiar with the legal basis of the case. That responsibility lies with the attorney. Still, you may want to become more familiar with the law because:

- You work in an area where you are frequently involved in legal processes.
- Knowledge is self-empowering.
- You can use your legal knowledge to explain certain information to your client.[15]
- You may feel less stress if you know what's happening.

---

[13]See Shuman and Sales (1998) for an excellent discussion of the concept of relevance and its application to expert witness testimony.

[14]Once again, there are important exceptions to the rule. For example, courts have considered "battered woman syndrome" as a valid defense for some women who have assaulted or killed abusive spouses.

[15]When providing an explanation of a legal concept to a client, remind your client that you are *not* providing a legal opinion. Refrain from providing any interpretation of law. Such behavior may be viewed as the unauthorized practice of law. Be safe and defer to your client's attorney.

- You may be able to work with the attorney on a more equal basis.
- You may become a more circumspect and effective witness once you understand the legal concepts about which you are testifying.
- You may prepare for testimony differently once you understand the legal concepts about which you are testifying.
- You may better assist the friendly attorney in preparing direct examination questions for you.
- You can better prepare for cross-examination and better understand the limitations of your testimony.

Becoming competent in an area of law is not easy, because it requires an understanding of the overall system, underlying principles and processes, as well as case law precedent and current rulings.

For a basic primer in law, you should refer to textbooks designed for psychiatrists, social workers, or other clinicians (such as Dickson, 1998; Salzman & Furman, 1998; Satterfield & Vayda, 1997; Swenson, 1997). University programs for these professionals frequently offer degree courses, continuing education courses, or seminars in law-related issues. The primary sources of law are statutes, regulations, and case law. However, these sources tend to be hard to access and difficult to understand if you are unfamiliar with "legalese." Law librarians and on-line services[16] are useful sources of information, should you need to do a search for relevant laws. Consolidations and pamphlets designed for nonattorneys may be available from government bookstores or agencies. Your agency could enlist an attorney or informed clinician to provide a seminar on a specific topic (e.g., human rights legislation and proceedings).

In preparing for a particular case, ask the attorney who intends to call you as a witness if there is certain legal information that you should have. He may be able to suggest particular sources of information, such as precedent cases, articles, videotapes, conferences, or seminars.

As a general framework of how to organize your learning about a legal issue, ask first for the *relevant legal principle*. Read about the principle and the various interpretations placed on the principle. Once you understand the principle, ask for information about *statutory obligations*. Ask for federal and state statutes on the topic. Digest their mean-

---

[16]See "Websites for Legal Research" in the References section.

ing. Integrate the meaning of the federal and state statutes with the general principle of law that you initially learned. Then, ask for specific *case law* that addresses the specific issues about which you are being asked to testify.

Many people find memorizing the principles and statutes to be more challenging than reading case law drawn from a state appellate or supreme court decision. The reason is that case law decisions tell a story, while legal principles are framed within historical precedents or legalistic theory. One learns law from case decisions through the narrative of the parties' competing stories. Behavioral science research suggests that people often recall more information and generally learn better from narrative than from almost any other form of teaching (Levinson, 1996). For many clinicians, once they learn the story that leads up to the court's decision, they are better able to recall the important aspects of the case that are relevant to their testimony.

Each witness's testimony may be viewed as a piece of a puzzle that the attorney is trying to present to the tribunal. Ask how your evidence fits into the bigger picture. Ask about the possible outcomes, desired outcomes, and likely outcomes of the hearing. Find out what evidence the case may turn upon. If the attorney says that you may not be allowed to know such information until after the trial, try to understand the attorney's reasoning.[17] Consider a divorce case in which Michael would be called to testify about his mediation with Philip and Paula.[18] Michael would be interested in why his testimony is significant and what types of orders the judge might fashion, depending on her findings. Initially Michael may think that the attorney wants him to testify about the access arrangements agreed to in mediation. However, from a legal perspective, the status quo may be more important than what is on paper. Accordingly, the attorney may want Michael to testify about the access arrangements that the parties told him were put into practice

---

[17]For example, Jon Gould was recently involved in a murder trial. His role was to conduct collateral interviews with people who knew the defendant. Jon was not provided with any information about any other aspect of the case. When asked about other aspects of the case during testimony, he could truthfully say that he had no knowledge beyond that of his limited role. It was frustrating to be outside of the informational loop about the case, but it was necessary to preserve the attorney's legal strategy.

[18]In many jurisdictions Michael would not be allowed to testify in his role as mediator except in very limited circumstances (e.g., to defend himself in a malpractice suite or if all parties agreed to waive any confidentiality or privilege for the mediation). For specific details in your own jurisdiction, check with your attorney and professional association.

rather than those to which they tentatively agreed. With knowledge of the real issues in the case, Michael can prepare more effectively.

Although it is important to have an understanding of what the actual laws say, it may also be important to understand how certain judges actually apply the laws. In family law, for example, some judges have been known to make custodial decisions based upon a "tender years doctrine" (i.e., that children under the tender age of 7 should be in the custody of their mothers) even though case law and statutory requirements have rejected this doctrine and state that decisions should be based upon the best interests of the particular child. Knowing the biases or decision-making history of a judge may help in creating a more effective legal strategy.

Facts and Theories

As a witness, your primary obligation is to answer questions as honestly as possible. If you are able to answer a question, do so. If you lack the knowledge to answer a question, then an honest answer is to admit that you do not know. You are not expected to know all of the facts of the case. You can enhance your value as a witness if you take time to review your information ahead of time, ensuring that you know what you are supposed to know. For example, if Freida were called to testify about her therapy with the Carveys, she should review her file and notes in advance of the hearing. This review will enable her to refresh her memory and organize her thoughts. While Freida may be able to use her notes at the hearing, her evidence will come across as more credible if she testifies from memory.

It may be useful to prepare a point-form summary of important facts that need to be presented. Share this summary with the friendly attorney and try to organize direct examination around those points. Do not try to memorize your testimony word-for-word, as you will not appear genuine and are likely to stumble through your answers.

In some cases you may be asked to gather specific types of facts for a hearing. For example, Evelyn may be asked to provide a family assessment, or Sam may be asked to assess Debra for exposure to maltreatment. Your information-gathering process must be thorough enough to withstand the rigors of cross-examination (see Chapter 5). If you qualify as an expert witness (Chapter 7), you must have a sound knowledge of the theory you used to assess or intervene in a particular case. To prepare for a case, review all literature on which you intend to rely during your testimony. Also, you should review and consider plausible *alternative* hypotheses that may be suggested by the data from your evaluation or treatment.[19] Be prepared to discuss the literature that supports the rival hypotheses and be able to present a cogent, logically consistent argument for your advocacy of one interpretation over another. If you intend to cite a particular study or reading, you may end up being tested about your knowledge of these sources in significant detail.

Since knowledge is limited to what you can recall, consider using strategies designed to enhance your memory. For example, in the ordinary course of practice, take notes during your interviews and leave time between sessions to reflect on each case. Use diagrams, pictures, or visualization (trying to picture a scene or image in your mind) to reinforce your memory. For example, Sam could use a genogram to graphically display the members of the Carvey family and the relationships between them. If you bring such graphic aids to court, make sure that you have enough copies to provide to each attorney and the judge. During your testimony, indicate that you have prepared a visual aid and offer that aid to the court. Do not hand anything to the judge. Simply state to the friendly attorney that you have available copies and would like to refer to the graphic during your testimony. There will likely be some discussion and/or examination of the document before it is handed to the judge. If there are no objections to its being presented to the judge, the friendly attorney will offer the document to the judge. If there are objections to its being handed to the judge, you may still continue to rely on it. However, no one else may be able to see it, and you may be called upon to provide more a detailed description of its usefulness since each party is not able to examine it for herself.

At the time of the hearing, ensure that you are well rested, relaxed, and sober, since fatigue, stress, and drugs can interfere with recall.

Skills

While clinicians are skilled at communication, the type of communication emphasized in clinical practice differs significantly from the type of

---

[19]According to the Specialty Guidelines for Forensic Psychologists (CEGFP, 1991), psychologists are ethically obliged to examine rival, plausible alternative hypotheses in order to provide the court with the most comprehensive set of information and opinions possible.

communication required in testifying. In delivering psychotherapy or other clinical services, the clinician facilitates the process, asks questions, and uses active listening skills. At a hearing, the attorney facilitates the process and asks questions, and the clinician uses information-providing skills. Whereas therapeutic interventions by clinicians generally occur in a private context in which the clinicians try to develop a safe environment for disclosure, a hearing is open to the public, and the atmosphere during cross-examination is adversarial.

Observation and practice are the primary means of preparing for the unique environment of a hearing. In addition to observing a live hearing, review educational videotapes or transcripts of similar hearings. Rehearsing testimony with your attorney is perhaps the best way to prepare. This type of preparation ensures that you will not be in the position of providing answers to questions that are beyond your knowledge. You cannot control the questions that are asked of you. The friendly attorney should be able to monitor the other attorney's questions and raise objections when inappropriate questions are posed.

The friendly attorney will likely not ask questions to which she does not already know the answer. The same is not true of the cross-examining attorney. Since opposing counsel has not prepared with you, it is likely that some questions will be posed which are outside the scope of proper examination. The cross-examining attorney is allowed to ask questions only about information that was brought up on direct examination. So, be careful not to open the door during cross-examination to a topic about which you have not offered testimony on direct examination.

A wonderful preparation experience is to role-play both the examination by your attorney and the cross-examination by the opposing attorney to prepare for the full range of possible questions. Role playing can reveal at least three important aspects of testimony. First, it can shed light on gaps in information and will guide you toward what additional information you need to gather prior to trial. Second, a role play will reveal inconsistencies in your testimony. Knowing how to present your information more consistently will add to the perception of you as a credible witness. Third, a role play in which you are being cross-examined will provide you with opportunities to learn how to deal with aggressive and maybe even unfair questioning techniques. For example, in a recent trial preparation Jon engaged in a role play where he was asked only yes and no questions. During the role play, the attorney was so successful at tying him up that Jon was unable to elaborate upon any aspect of his information except that which could be answered by yes or no. Each time he attempted to explain his reasoning, the attorney would yell, "Your Honor, the witness is nonresponsive to the question!" The objection was sustained, and Jon was told to answer only the precise questions he was asked. His responses were limited to "Yes" or "No." It was maddeningly frustrating!

In this example Jon was role-playing with a friendly attorney, who in fact was also a friend. Once the attorney stepped into the role of cross-examining attorney, Jon indicated he found himself feeling genuine disdain and anger, despite the fact it was a role play! The strong feelings that were aroused during the role play helped Jon to prepare for testifying more effectively even while feeling strongly negative feelings toward the questioner.

The attorney can coach you about how to streamline testimony, organize relevant material, and articulate clearly. Some clinicians wonder whether it is appropriate for an attorney to tell them how to testify. Ethically an attorney is permitted to help a witness with the *manner of testifying* but should not direct the witness about *what to say*. The line can be fuzzy, such as when an attorney suggests certain wording that has slightly different connotations. During trial preparation, Sam uses the word "mistreatment," but Lori suggests that he substitute the word "abuse." Sam should ask about the significance of this change. To test whether you should adopt a suggestion, there are two things to consider. The first is whether the reframed statement accurately reflects the meaning as well as context of your original statement. You must feel comfortable that your response would be honest and accurate. A second concern is whether your statement properly reflects the literature. That is, are you using terms that are consistent with how mental health professionals use the terms? For example, do you know if spanking a 3-year-old child twice on his bottom is a reasonable discipline response by a parent to a young child's transgressions. The attorney may want you to talk about the father's alleged physical abuse of the child since such a characterization might help the mother's argument for relocation. Do you label this as abuse? Do you label it as maltreatment? Do you describe the research on the use of spanking with young children?

Begin with the presumption that the attorney will (1) act in good faith and (2) present an argument that most favors her client's position. Be prepared for occasions when you will be faced with an ethical conundrum. If you have evidence that runs contrary to a client's case, the attorney is more likely to pass you over as a witness than to ask you to testify and lie. An attorney is ethically permitted to suggest what to emphasize and what points to answer only if asked. It is not ethical for an attorney to knowingly lead false evidence or to ask you to distort or suppress evidence. Your options for such requests include complying with the attorney, consulting with the law society or your professional association, and speaking with your attorney. If an attorney discovers that she has unintentionally led misleading evidence, she also has a duty to rectify the misunderstanding with the court and opposing counsel.

For clinicians, honesty is a professional value. However, some clinicians place other values ahead of honesty. Radical clinicians, for example, may be willing to lie to protect a client or to advance a greater social cause (e.g., a clinician who supports euthanasia may lie to protect a person who assists in a suicide, even though this is illegal). Be aware of the potential consequences—for you, your client, and others—in order to make an informed decision.[20]

For those who place personal rather than professional values, ethics, and behavior at the top of the list, it is important to recognize two important aspects of these choices. First, driving a personal agenda in a court of law under the guise of a professional view hurts all clinical professionals involved in the system. The system learns to mistrust those who disingenuously represent themselves as representing their profession yet push a personal agenda without clearly articulating to the court that their expressed views are not a reflection of their profession.

Second, representing one's personal agenda to the court as if it were a professional agenda may be, at its core, an immoral action founded upon deception and/or omission. As Lavin and Sales (1998) eloquently describe, the moral foundation of mental health expert witness testimony is an allegiance to a truthful representation of the research, the ethics, and the clinical experiences that inform our decision making. A moral advocacy position would be based upon an accurate representation to the court that the information being presented represents a per-

---

[20]For an outline of the consequences, see Footnote 7, this chapter.

sonal rather than a professional agenda. It would acknowledge that only one side of an argument is being presented rather than informing the court of rival, plausible alternative points of view and their reasoning.

If you choose to advocate for one side of an issue, it is ethically appropriate to let the court know that this is how you are presenting your arguments. This lets the court know that, regardless of how compelling your argument, you are not presenting a comprehensive view of a particular controversy. Alternatively, you could present alternate sides of an argument and then indicate your opinion to the court, based on all of the reasoning you have analyzed and presented.

If you have a practical understanding of legal processes, you may be able to help the attorney strategize. For example, Evelyn has presented evidence before a particular judge on numerous occasions. She can suggest what type of presentation tends to be most persuasive to this judge and what type of argument falls on deaf ears. Freida used to work for the human rights tribunal and knows that they prefer to resolve issues through negotiation. Following trial preparation, Michael identified significant issues that he did not have an opportunity to address. He suggested that Lori ask certain questions to afford him this opportunity. Together they created a list of questions, identified the order in which they would be asked, and each carried a copy of the questions into the courtroom. Lori used her list for direct examination.

Unfortunately, rehearsing is an area of preparation often neglected by attorneys. If you want more intensive preparation than the attorney calling you as a witness is willing to provide, you can practice on your own or with a colleague who is knowledgeable about testifying. Practicing in front of a mirror or using videotape can help you to reflect on your total presentation. Focus on your physical positioning when you talk. Listen for your tonal quality. Consider appropriate eye contact both with the judge and jury as well as the attorneys. Wait patiently for each question to be completely posed and for any possible objection to the question. Then, examine how you respond both to friendly as well as challenging questions. Look for consistency in your response style. Look for the appearance of openness and honesty. The best testifying advice we have ever received is to be perceived as transparent. The message you want to communicate is that you have nothing to hide. You want to convey the message that you know what you know and that there are many things you do not know, many things you may have done differently if different information had been presented to you. You want to convey the message that you are open to being wrong, yet you did the best you could with what you had at the time you did it.

Determine the type of image you want to convey to the decision makers, for example, objectivity, alliance with the disadvantaged, sympathy, or expertise. Different images may be desirable for different cases. How you present yourself should reflect the image you have decided to portray, from how you dress to how you speak and gesture. Consider how to develop a style that works best for you. For example, Michael may be naturally rational and subdued. A highly passionate presentation may not come across as genuine for him. He will have little problem coming across as thoughtful and reliable. He will have to ensure that he does not appear too distant or abstract.

MENTAL PREPARATION

One of the most common concerns among clinicians called to testify is the anxiety that it provokes. Stress can derive from a range of sources: not knowing what to expect; fear of looking bad on the stand; anxiety about public speaking; or lack of confidence in your abilities as a witness. Label your fears and determine what type of preparation is needed.

Observing hearings and role playing will help you to become familiar and comfortable with the process. Feel free to ask your attorney "dumb questions." She will appreciate having an informed witness rather than someone who feigns wisdom. Find out how long you will be on the stand[21] and how grueling it might be. Ask about the worst-case scenario. Michael might think that his mediation skills will be put into question. Lori can reassure him that his competence is not a relevant issue and that is not why he is being called to testify. If his competence were likely to be called into question, Lori and Michael could strategize

---

[21]To be safe, multiply the attorney's estimate for time on the stand by two. Although her direct examination may be 30 minutes, you may be cross-examined for a longer period of time. Often, the more important your testimony is to the case, the longer the period of cross-examination. Also, allot time for possible redirect and recross-examinations.

about how to deal with this possibility. Some witnesses fear that they will get burned in cross-examination; however, cases are won or lost on the facts of the case. Your best protection is to be aware of the facts and speak honestly. Most examinations are dry affairs. Surprise testimony and witnesses breaking down on the stand are only common on television and in the movies. Prepare yourself with positive self-messages for when you take the stand: "I am not on trial. I am a competent clinician. I can get through this as long as I remain calm. And I have nothing to hide."

Make use of universal strategies for dealing with stress, such as a proper diet, good physical health and activity, rest, breathing exercises, visualization, and taking breaks from other stressful activities. Use your support network and build in additional support. Because of the potential for embarrassment, some people tend to withdraw socially when they are embroiled in a legal conflict. Consider whom you can rely on for support without breaching the client's right to confidentiality.

Plan ahead for what you will do in the final hour or so before you testify. Having explicit relaxing exercises or planning to review specific materials prior to testifying can reduce feelings of anxiety during this time (Brodsky, 1991). As part of your final preparation, ensure that you are well rested and mentally alert. Be selective about what you eat and drink so that you do not become "gassy" or require frequent restroom breaks. Avoid the use of drugs as relaxants since they tend to affect memory and recall.

PREPARING YOUR CLIENTS

In addition to preparing yourself for a hearing, consider whether you need to take steps to ensure that your client is also prepared. The attorney calling you as a witness might ask you not to speak with your client before a hearing to avoid conflicts or other legal complications. Even in such cases, you may have an ethical obligation to ensure that the client has access to another clinician or an alternative support system. Discuss your ethical obligations both with the attorney and with the client. Make sure that any referral you make for your client does not compromise your relationship with the attorney. Make sure that your relationship with the attorney does not compromise your ethical responsibility to your client.

For clinical reasons, you and your client should discuss the impact of your acting as a witness on your relationship with your client. Let the client know that you will be a witness and be honest about what you will say to the tribunal. If a conflict exists between the client and yourself, acknowledge the existence of the conflict and the difficulties of being involved in a legal process. Empathize with the client's feelings of anger, frustration, disbelief, sadness, or betrayal. You may find that disclosing negative information to a client in a frank manner can lead to positive changes. If Freida plans to testify about Philip's limitations as a parent, Philip can take steps to deal with these limitations. A client may change his behavior to try to influence your testimony and recommendations. You may be concerned that confronting a client in this manner infringes on a client's right to self-determination. Consider, however, whether it would be less of an infringement to wait until the hearing for the client to hear your information or recommendations.

If you are in a forensic role (such as Evelyn is, in her role as the court's evaluator for the custodial assessment), then you may be prohibited from sharing the report with each parent. If you are in doubt about whether you can share the report, check with the court. If you are in a clinical treatment role, you should not be in a position of preparing a report for the court unless the parties have agreed in advance or there is a court order for treatment that includes reporting responsibilities to the court. In cases where you have both treatment and reporting roles, it is generally appropriate to review your written report with the parties prior to submitting the report to the court.

If you are in a clinical role and you have prepared a report to submit to an attorney, you may wish to talk with your client as well as the attorney about the contents of the report. In addition to dealing with feelings, your client may need to rethink whether to proceed to a hearing. The manner in which you present your report can either encourage settlement or aggravate the level of conflict (Chisholm & McNaughton, 1990). Let the client know your understanding of how your report will be used in the hearing. Advise your client to talk with her attorney about how your report is expected to be used. Then, if appropriate and legally permissible, you need to be open to the client's right to dispute your report's contents. The client may be able to provide suggestions for how to reword the document to make it less embarrassing or troubling.

If your client works with you to reword some of the information, be prepared to defend your reasons for allowing the client to influence you as well as your reasons for allowing the client to change the words that reflect your professional judgment. Such challenges often focus on your lack of certainty, your alliance with the client rather than alliance with the truth, and your apparent bias in favor of your client. The bottom line is that your credibility will be challenged, making it appear that you have sold out your professional integrity to protect your client. Whether this is a fair representation or not, it is an often-used attack on your decision to allow your client to change your work product.

Remember that your client may not know the legal implications of including or excluding certain information and may need to be referred for legal advice. Although you may be hesitant to be the messenger of bad news, your report is more likely to have a harmful impact if your client first learns of its contents from her attorney, from filed documents, or at the hearing, rather than from you directly.

In fact, an argument can be made that as a treating clinician, your report about your client needs first to be discussed with the client before being forwarded to the attorney. This is because your client holds the privilege of the communication and allows you to release information to others only upon informed consent. Your client cannot provide informed consent if you have not first discussed the contents of the communication with her! Therefore, if you are in a treatment role, you should always discuss with your client what you intend to release and how it will be worded prior to its release. Anything less is likely not informed consent and may place you in an ethical as well as legal conundrum. You should also inform your client that, should the case go to trial, you do not have control over the questions asked and the types of information that you may be required to divulge while testifying.

You may be able to downplay the adversarial aspects of an adjudication. Freida, Paula, and Philip are all concerned about Debra's best interests. All of them want the judge to make a fair decision. Freida could explain to Philip that they have an honest difference of opinion about what is best for Debra and that an impartial judge can help them decide what to do. Avoid becoming entrenched in a particular position. As a clinician, you do not have a personal interest in a specific outcome. You are presenting the best information you have to help an adjudicator make the best decision possible.

You may be able to provide information about the hearing process, but be careful not to provide the client with legal advice. Ensure that your client has been advised to obtain counsel if she needs guidance or representation and remember to record your advice in your treatment notes, complete with the date you discussed the issue and your client's stated position. Once the client obtains counsel, record the name and address of the attorney in your records. If your client refuses your advice, record in your notes the reasons why and consult with a colleague and/or an attorney about how best to handle any current or future requests for your treatment notes.

In some cases you may believe your client should not be present at a hearing because of the negative psychological impact on him. For example, a client who is suicidal may be pushed into crisis if she were exposed to testimony about the manner in which she was sexually assaulted. If you are concerned about the impact of your testimony on your client, you may be able to adjust the manner of your presentation rather than try to exclude your client from the hearing. You may be faced with a dilemma if altering your testimony to protect your client detracts from your ability to be open and honest as a witness. Some clinicians are overly protective of their clients or underestimate the possibility of positive therapeutic impact of exposing a client to difficult information. A survivor of sexual abuse may actually benefit from sitting through a trial, so long as she has sufficient preparation and support.

If you harbor such concerns about your client's ability to be exposed to your testimony, raise this issue with her attorney. You may also need to consider whether your testimony will adversely affect or fatally injure your relationship with your client. Should these issues present themselves, consult a colleague or your attorney for advice.

Another area to discuss with your client is what will happen after the hearing. Can you resume your clinical relationship? Does the client want to be referred to another clinician? Can you help the client to deal with various potential outcomes? In some cases clinicians are helpful in implementing the terms of a court decision (e.g., supervising terms of access, providing assessment or therapeutic services, or monitoring implementation). Most tribunals do not have the power to order a person to attend counseling. However, if you discuss the possibility of clinical intervention with a client in advance, the client may agree to a consent order that specifies that the client will attend psychotherapy sessions.

Make sure that any directive you receive from the court clearly indicates your reporting responsibilities. If you are to provide treatment updates to the court, make sure that there is sufficient information in the court's order about how such communications are to occur. If you are to provide treatment to the client and provide no information to the court, it may be wise to have the order specify that the litigant (rather than the court) is your client. In this way, issues of privilege and confidentiality are clearly established in the order.

Chapter 5

Oral Testimony at an Adjudication

If you are thinking, "Halfway through the book and you're just getting to the hearing?" you should consider how long it takes in real life to get this far. If you have just started reading the book here because you will be in court tomorrow, you may have missed some important information and should probably go back to Chapter 1. It could be a late night. . . . Irrespective of how you arrived here, the purposes of this chapter are to familiarize you with what to expect at a hearing and to provide guidance for testifying. We begin by describing the examination-in-chief, more commonly called the direct examination. We then present our "Top 10 Hard-and-Fast Rules for Witnesses." As will become readily apparent as you read on, even hard-and-fast rules can be soft and slow. We will then take you through the process of cross-examination and provide suggestions for how to deal with difficult situations.

This chapter provides a repertoire of strategies from which you can draw. Rather than follow them by rote, consider the underlying reasons for each suggestion and whether these reasons apply in your situation. This process is similar to the use of microskills, intentional interviewing, or ethnosensitive practice (Ivey & Ivey, 1999). Each tribunal has a unique culture. When a reflective clinician enters work with people from another culture, she takes responsibility for adjusting her use of self in order to present in a culturally appropriate manner through control of her verbal and body language. As you decide how to present yourself at a hearing, consider your role and the purpose of the hearing.

To simplify the discussion, we will focus on a clinician who is called to testify about her observations while working with a client, leaving the discussion of opinion evidence and expert testimony to Chapter 7. The clinician's primary role is to present her evidence in a factually accurate and credible manner. You may have additional intentions and will adjust your presentation accordingly.

To appear credible, you need to decide upon the best way to demonstrate candor, impartiality, trustworthiness, respectfulness, expert knowledge, and confidence. For example, honesty may be demonstrated by steady speech, consistent messages, and poised body language. Fidgeting, shifting your eyes, contradicting yourself, and perspiring may be perceived as signs of dishonesty. However, in different arenas or with different decision makers, you may need to adjust your manner of presentation. Direct eye contact in some cultures is a sign of attentiveness; in other cultures, it is a sign of disrespect. Just as different ethnic groups operate with different cultural norms, so do different legal systems or different courtrooms within the same jurisdiction.

Think about your audience and, in particular, the decision maker(s) at the hearing. What type of information will be most persuasive to this audience—scientific facts, emotional appeals, anecdotal information, moral arguments, or information that has the support of a larger group (e.g., a petition or endorsement from a professional group)? How can you present yourself in a manner that is most effective? Effectiveness as a witness depends on total presentation of the person including preparation, knowledge of relevant material, dress, appearance, speech, style, and confidence. Some decision makers will be impressed by one style, whereas other decision makers will be impressed by another.

DIRECT EXAMINATION

As we noted in Chapter 1, the direct examination is conducted by the attorney who calls the witness to testify. In general, this attorney cannot suggest specific answers to his questions. The reason for this rule is to avoid allowing an attorney to put words in the witness's mouth. Further, this attorney cannot impugn his own witness.[1]

---

[1]"Impugn" refers to attacking the credibility of a witness or calling her testimony into question.

These rules of direct examination have three primary exceptions. First, attorneys are given latitude to ask leading questions to guide a witness quickly through uncontroversial issues: "Your name is Michael Elliot?" "You are a mediator with Elliot and Associates?" "You were hired by the Carveys to mediate the terms of custody and access with their daughter?"

The second exception concerns "hostile witnesses." Attorneys usually call witnesses who are either neutral or sympathetic to their clients' interests. In some situations, an attorney will call a witness who is adverse in interest. If the tribunal deems the witness hostile, then the attorney conducting the direct examination will be permitted to ask questions as if it were a cross-examination (discussed below).

A third exception relevant to clinicians is that someone appointed by the court to provide an assessment may be cross-examined by both parties.

Since an attorney calling you as a witness should have discussed his questions and your testimony with you ahead of time, the direct examination should be relatively straightforward and free of surprises.[2] Starting with a direct examination gives you time to feel comfortable on the stand. If your evidence were entered into the court record solely through documents, you would not have time to get acclimated to testifying before being subjected to difficult and hostile questions in cross-examination.

An examination usually begins with questions about who you are and how you came to have information relevant to the case. Following these introductions, the attorney leads you through your story, typically in chronological order. The friendly attorney will focus primarily on evidence in support of her case. However, the attorney may also ask questions that raise evidence contrary to her case, knowing that such evidence will likely come out in cross-examination anyway.

While some judges and tribunals are passive, others ask their own questions during either the direct examination or the cross-examination. Show them the same respect you do other questioners. You do not have to agree with the suggestions put forward in a judge's questions. However, such questions may be particularly important because they indicate the focus of the decision-makers' interest. Their questions also give

---

[2]During this stage, witnesses are more likely to surprise an attorney with new information, rather than an attorney surprising the witness with a fresh question. Either type of surprise should be avoided.

you the opportunity to help them with the information they need to make a particular decision.

It is appropriate to provide information counter to a judge's belief. For example, a judge may ask a question that suggests a poor understanding of current research. Recently a judge asked about the potential harm to a 5-year-old in having overnight visitation with her father. The expert was able to point to three recent research articles that helped the judge to see how his ideas about overnight visitations as harmful were not supported by current research. Whether such testimony was able to affect the judge's personal bias about such decisions is another story and an important question to keep in mind. You might be able to teach the judge something new about current research or treatment techniques. However, that does not mean that the new knowledge will change the judge's strongly held personal beliefs.

TEN RULES OF TESTIFYING

The following 10 rules apply regardless of who is asking the questions.

Rule 1: Tell the Truth, the Whole Truth, and Nothing but the Truth

Honesty is the most basic rule of giving evidence as well as a legal commitment you make by giving an oath. Although telling the truth seems so basic that no explanation is needed, be aware of certain traps. In particular, when you are asked a question, you may feel obliged to answer in a way that will reflect well on yourself or your client. After all, if the attorney asks you a question, he must think that you have a good answer. However, honesty may require admitting that you do not have one. *If you do not know the answer to a question, say so. If you do not remember the information requested, say so.* It is better to appear ignorant or admit to having an imperfect memory than to be caught trying to cover up what you really do not know. On the other hand, do not say "I don't know" or "I don't remember" just to avoid a difficult or embarrassing question.

Be forthright about evidence that goes against your preferred case. Do not feel obliged to rationalize damaging facts or to show reluctance to concede a point in favor of opposing counsel. A short answer may be better than a long explanation because it will downplay the importance attributed to the answer. Sam might admit, "Yes, Philip has been cooperative with my investigation," even though this may argue against Sam's belief that Debra is in need of protective services.

Testify about what you observed even if it does not conform to other testimony that has been presented. Different people can have different observations, perceptions, and memories. It is up to the tribunal rather than the witness to reconcile these differences. The other person may be wrong. You may want to discuss discrepancies with your attorney outside of the hearing and after you have completed your testimony. Talking about your testimony during a break is inappropriate. Once you take the stand, you should not talk about your testimony except when being questioned.

A troubling situation may arise if your client or another witness testifies about something that you know to be untrue. During your testimony, focus on the facts and information you have, as well as the basis for these facts. Rather than testify that the other person is lying, establish the truth of your version.

Certainly there may be situations where a witness comes across as not completely honest. As a professional clinician, do not let unconscious biases creep into your testimony. If Freida feels sympathetic toward Paula, Freida may exaggerate evidence in Paula's favor or downplay evidence against her. Freida's testimony that "Paula provided *all* of Debra's parenting" could be an innocent embellishment that hurts Freida's credibility and sets her up for cross-examination. If Freida is asked if she is biased toward Paula, Freida may be tempted to say that she is objective and nonjudgmental. On the other hand, it may be more honest for Freida to admit that, yes, she does like Paula as a person and thinks she has demonstrated many positive parenting skills. By admitting her sympathies in a manner appropriate to her clinical role, Freida maintains her credibility more than if she denied that she possessed any prejudices.

There are times when you may be tempted to stray from the absolute truth. As the authors of this text, we cannot condone lying under oath. If you are tempted to stray from the truth, be sure to consider the potentially dire consequences of doing so—as well as alternative means of achieving the same objective. We firmly believe that, if people think through the consequences and alternatives carefully, they will be more likely to be honest.

Rule 2: Convey Professionalism

If you are called to testify in your professional capacity as a clinician, consider what type of presentation may be expected of you. Typically, professionalism implies formality, competence, and objectivity.

Although you should avoid overdramatizing, professionalism need not rule out your testifying in a warm and interesting manner. Use your public speaking skills to convey your information in an engaging manner, for example, by using inflections in your voice, vivid language, and personalized testimony. Your testimony will have little impact if the decision maker falls asleep during your delivery of it.

It is also appropriate to advocate for a position forcefully, provided that you have a solid research or clinical foundation for such advocacy. Such advocacy may also best be presented by offering alternative rival positions and then explaining how the current data are best interpreted through the position *you* advocate.

Rule 3: Respect the Formalities of the Tribunal

Legal processes tend to be staid and rational proceedings with comparatively few theatrics. Legal professionals and witnesses are inclined to dress conservatively[3] as a sign of respect for the solemnity of the process and the serious issues at stake. Although tribunals vary greatly in their formality, all legal processes have rituals. Many court rituals revolve around how to show respect for the judge. While the designation of judges differs among courts, in general, judges in most courts are addressed as "Your Honor." If in doubt, "Judge" is generally acceptable. Respect for judges is demonstrated by standing when a judge addresses you, when she walks into the room, or when she gets up to leave. Decorum tends to be less formal when the hearing is not conducted by a public court judge. Mr. and Ms. are usually the favored forms of address for other people, such as the attorneys or parties to an action. Entering or leaving the hearing while it is in session may be prohibited. A final rule of respect is to avoid arguing or flagrantly disagreeing with the decision maker.

---

[3]Although you may need to dress conservatively, also try to dress comfortably. This will enable you to look and feel comfortable and confident, and you will also be able to focus more intently on the substance of your testimony.

Many rules in hearings are the same as those learned in kindergarten (Fulghum, 1988): play fair, don't hit people, no speaking when it's not your turn; no gum or food; no joking around; ask for a brief recess if you have to go to the washroom; and take off your hat when you come inside. While the rules should be taken seriously, there are some exceptions that your kindergarten teacher might not have accepted: passing notes discreetly; drinking water during your testimony; using humor to make a point (occasionally and respectfully); and donning religious head wear, such as yarmulkes or turbans.

When you are asked to take the witness stand, sit properly. Do not swivel or rotate in the chair, nor rock back and forth. Try not to move about needlessly. Look at the attorney asking the questions and then provide your answers either to the judge, the jury, or the attorney. If the witness chair is bolted to the floor, you may need to lean forward to place your documents on a desk or platform.

Rule 4: Speak Slowly, Loudly, and without Hesitation

Ensure that your speech is given slowly enough for the tribunal recorder and others to record your testimony accurately and completely. Consider spelling unusual names and words to help those taking notes or recording your testimony. Your pacing may depend upon the conceptual difficulty of your information and the nature of your audience, but is generally slower than normal conversation. Pause briefly before answering a question to allow the other attorney time to register any objections and to give yourself a moment to think about how to articulate your answer. If you need time to think, take control by saying, "Let me consider my answer for a moment." Then take a moment to formulate your response. If you need more time, you could ask for a moment more to think. Taking the extra time demonstrates that you are taking the question seriously. Some witnesses use covert ways to buy time to think, for example, by asking the attorney to repeat or rephrase the question, dropping a paper clip and reaching down to pick it up, or providing information that does not really answer the question. Such strategies may work but can be distracting or might suggest that you are trying to avoid the question. Pausing too long or too often may appear as uncertainty or insincerity. Clear and fluid speech tends to impart greater confidence in what you are saying. This does not mean you have to give the perfect speech, since perfect speech may sound overrehearsed and also lack credibility.

Anxiety may lead a person to hurry his answers. If you feel pressured into answering, take a deep breath and answer at a comfortable pace. Most legal proceedings are very methodical. The tribunal will not expect you to rush your responses.

Gauge your volume to be loud enough to be heard by everyone in the room. If you will be using a microphone, practice with one ahead of time to become familiar with the optimal volume and distance from the microphone. You may also need to talk into a microphone that is for recording purposes rather than amplification.

Rule 5: Provide Clear and Concise Answers

Attorneys usually advise their witnesses not to volunteer unnecessary information, make speeches, or go off on tangents. Brief answers enable the attorney calling you to lay a foundation of information to build a case. Keeping your answers short may also prevent you from getting into trouble by saying something you will regret during cross-examination.

Closed-ended questions can often be answered with a simple "Yes," "No," or "That is not what I observed." Avoid indefinite terms such as "From what I can remember," "So far as I know," or "I guess so." These comments put unnecessary qualifications on your answers and weaken the impact of your testimony. Handling a yes/no question with a negative in it can be tricky. "Didn't you screen your client for suicidal ideation?" A simple yes or no answer is ambiguous. A preferred answer would be "Yes, I did screen" or "No, I did not screen." Be careful about questions that contain double negatives such as "Is it not true that you did not attend the movies that night." Rather than a "Yes" or "No" response, we encourage a more complete sentence, such as "Yes, I did attend the movie that night."

Gear the level of your language to your audience. When the decision makers are professionals from your field of clinical practice, then technical, professional language is appropriate. But when the decision makers are unfamiliar with the jargon used in your profession, then scrupulously avoid its use. If you need to use technical language, be prepared to provide definitions of your terms in plain language. If you use a lot of psychobabble, some people will view your artful obscureness as detracting from the importance of your testimony—as well as your credibility.

Colloquialisms and slang not only detract from professionalism but also may have ambiguous meanings. However, if you are asked to quote what a client said in your presence, do not be embarrassed if you need to use obscene language.

Be careful about speaking through the use of gestures or body language (e.g., nodding yes or no). People may be unable to see your gestures, and it is hard to record nonverbal responses. If you do answer with a gesture, the attorney may describe your gesture so that it is included in the transcript of the hearing. Rather than saying, "It was this big . . . " and holding your hands out to demonstrate, describe the size in inches, centimeters, or other standard measures. Gestures and changes in the volume of your voice can be used to emphasize points and to make your testimony sound more interesting, but they should not be used to change the meaning of your testimony. In print, "Yeah, sure" is recorded as total agreement—even if you intended to say it *sarcastically*.

Even though the "hard-and-fast rule" says to keep it brief, occasional elaboration on key points can significantly strengthen your testimony. The extent to which you can recall detail indicates the quality of your memory and the accuracy of your testimony. Freida's recollection of important sessions with the Carveys will naturally carry greater weight, for example, if she can accurately place them by specific dates, times, and locations. You will have to decide when it is advantageous to be concise and when it is preferable to provide greater detail.

Rule 6: Let the Attorney Lead the Questions

During examinations, attorneys are responsible for asking the questions and witnesses are responsible for answering them. Because clinicians are used to facilitating communication, they often find this division of roles to be stifling. It is hard to resist helping out an attorney by providing information that you think is important, regardless of the question asked. Yet, you may be rebuked for trying to lead the examination in a different direction. The time to work together with the attorney on the line of questioning is during preparation. Once you are on the stand, allow the attorney to maintain control of the interviewing process. During preparation, you may ask the attorney to provide you with some open-ended questions, such as "Do you have any other important information you wish to add?"

Answer all questions unless one of the attorneys states an objection that is upheld by the tribunal. If you start to provide an answer and one of the attorneys states an objection, pause until the matter has been discussed and ruled upon. Once said, a statement has lasting impact, regardless of whether the tribunal rules the evidence inadmissible. As a witness, do not participate in the discussion between attorneys about whether the information should be admitted, so that you appear neutral. On occasion, you may be asked to leave the hearing while the objection is discussed. This procedure ensures that your evidence is not tainted by the debate over admissibility. You have no need to worry if you are asked to leave. After the attorneys make their arguments concerning the objection, the tribunal will either ask you to answer the question or ask the attorney to go on to other questions.

If you have rehearsed the direct examination, be careful about anticipating questions. Listen carefully to each question and ensure that you understand it before answering. The attorney may decide to vary the line of questioning from how it was originally rehearsed.

Rule 7: Just the Facts, Ma'am/Sir

The primary role of most witnesses is to testify about facts. Only witnesses who qualify as experts can provide opinion evidence. Accordingly, if you are called as a fact witness, focus on concrete, observable, and specific information. Consider if Freida were asked about what she observed when she met with Debra. To say "Debra was traumatized" involves an interpretation or opinion. If Freida were asked just to provide facts, she could describe the actions and events that led her to her conclusions, all without explicitly stating her opinion: "Debra became silent when I asked about her father. She ran to the corner of the room and covered herself with a blanket."

Avoid language with subjective interpretations. "The meeting was long" could mean 10 minutes or 10 hours, depending on whose perspective you consider. Use objective measures wherever possible.

Sticking to the facts does not mean that your testimony should be dry or uninteresting. Consider the use of language that will have an intellectual or emotional impact. Use descriptive language that enables the decision maker to better visualize the events being described. Rather than saying "Philip's house was a mess," describe the stench of the beer in the carpets, the fuzzy blue mold inside the refrigerator, and the unlaundered clothes strewn across the living room.

Rule 8: Keep Your Composure

Use the anxiety reduction strategies we described in Chapter 4 to remain cool and collected during your testimony (e.g., self talk, taking a deep breath). While difficulties in maintaining your composure are most likely to arise during cross-examination, you may also be confronted by difficult questions during the direct examination. Attorneys as a whole suggest that you should not take such confrontation personally, since each attorney is just playing his or her role in an intentionally adversarial process. Regardless of their intentions, you may feel that you are being unfairly attacked. Unfortunately, if your response is overly defensive—demonstrating testiness or outright hostility—some decision makers may construe such defensiveness as a sign of a lack of integrity, certainty, or professionalism on your part. Avoid defensive responses that will hurt your credibility such as hedging, stalling, arguing with the questioner, sounding overly apologetic, raising your voice, speaking over the questioner, or providing rationalizations for mistakes or omissions. You might try a matter-of-fact response, such as "Yes, I did not find out whether this client was eligible for social assistance. In hindsight, obtaining such information would have been a useful step." On the other hand wisecracks and sarcasm are totally inappropriate. For example, "No, I am not a quack psychiatrist—but thank you for asking" sounds both unprofessional and petty. Leave out the crack about "thank you for asking"—sarcasm inevitably backfires.

Maintaining your composure does not imply that your testimony should lack all emotion. If Freida were defending the efficacy of her therapy, describing her interventions in a rational manner would doubtless be best. If she were challenged about her concern for Debra, however, her emotions might naturally be evidenced in describing the effects of abuse on Debra.

Although you may not be permitted to have a break just because you are facing difficult questions, there are some situations where you can ask for a break in order to regain your composure, such as if you are tired, not feeling well, or need to use the washroom. Tribunals are reluctant to interrupt the flow of testimony due to a belief that honest responses are more likely if you have to respond immediately. If you are in the midst of a key sequence of questions, the tribunal will call for a break only if you are in acute discomfort.

Rule 9: Maintain Eye Contact

Some attorneys recommend that you maintain eye contact primarily with the person asking questions, while others suggest that you provide your testimony directly to the judge or jury. Occasional glances at your client or at other parties in the room may make your presentation seem more natural, so long as these glances are not overlong or distracting. If you peer intently at your attorney when answering another person's questions, you will look as though you are being coached.

Rule 10: Use Notes to Refresh Your Memory

Ideally, you have a perfect memory and can accurately recall any information you are asked. In the real world, you cannot remember every contact you had with a particular client over the past 10 months, and perhaps not even what you had for breakfast today. If you maintain good clinical records (as outlined in Chapter 6), you may be able to use them during your oral testimony.

If you want to use your notes during a court proceeding, ask the judge, "May I refer to my notes to refresh my memory?" The judge may ask the following questions to qualify your notes: "Are these your own notes? When were these notes made? Were the events still fresh in your memory when you made these notes? Since you made these notes, have you made any additions or deletions?" Ideally, you can answer honestly that the notes were yours, you made them immediately following your contact with the client based on notes taken during the session, the events were still fresh in your memory, and you have not made any changes to the notes. The judge will allow you to use your notes to refresh your memory, provided that you made the notes contemporaneously with the events recorded and that you are using the notes only to refresh your memory rather than to replace information that you do not currently remember. You must also be prepared to provide the relevant notes or file to the court. Bring originals and several copies. Noncourt tribunals are generally less strict about the preconditions for using notes.

The primary advantage of using your notes is that you can check for details such as dates and times. Providing such details can enhance your credibility and demonstrate that you have maintained an accurate record of events. The main disadvantage of relying on your notes is that, once you refresh your memory or introduce any part of your notes, you may be cross-examined on all of the notes in your record. You may also waive any privilege. During preparation, review your notes with the cooperating attorney to determine whether they are complete, accurate, and able to withstand cross-examination. You can then decide whether using your notes is a good idea.

If you decide to use your notes, do not rely too much on them, since this may indicate that you do not have a current memory. Reading notes also tends to be monotonous and uninteresting. If you are able to answer questions accurately without notes, your testimony will tend to be more persuasive. If you can give more precise answers by using your notes, however, doing so adds to the credibility of your answers.

Using notes to refresh your memory is distinctly different from entering documentary evidence (including notes) into the record of the hearing. If you use notes just to refresh your memory, then only your oral testimony goes into the record. If your notes are entered as an exhibit, then they also form part of the official record of the hearing.

CROSS-EXAMINATION

The purposes of cross-examination are to test the reliability, accuracy, and credibility of testimony provided in the direct examination. The attorney can also try to bring out additional information favorable to his client.

During cross-examination, the attorney may ask leading questions, suggest answers, and impugn the witness. Since it involves such risks, cross-examination is the aspect of legal proceedings that clinicians fear most. After all, clinicians can occasionally be made to look derelict or incompetent during that phase of the proceeding. You might even mess up a case for your client. But remember, pitchers give batters too much credit. You can psyche yourself out and create more problems for yourself than anything the attorney can possibly conjure up. If you are honest, relaxed, and prepared, the risks entailed in cross-examination are low. If you provide a solid direct examination, the opposing attorney will have little to cross-examine. Prior to the hearing, your attorney can help you identify the likely focus of cross-examination and prepare you to respond most effectively.

Try to think of cross-examination as a safety check that helps to ensure that your evidence is thorough and correct (Landau, Wolfson, Landau, Bartoletti, & Mesbur, 2000). You would not want the court to operate on false or faulty information. Clinicians are not opposed in principle to safety checks (e.g., the use of second opinions in clinical diagnoses and interrater reliability checks in social research). It is natural to feel some anxiety during cross-examination. Few people really enjoy it, but the risks of cross-examination should not be blown out of proportion. The vast majority of cases are won or lost on the facts rather than one witness's performance on the stand. If you have strong facts, it may even be impossible to blunder badly enough to lose the case.

We will take you through a number of different tactics that you *might* face in cross-examination. Do not be overly concerned. These are for demonstration purposes only—to help you to prepare for the worst. Cross-examination can also be risky for the cross-examining attorney, since many of these tactics can backfire. After all, litigation attorneys are trained not to ask a question unless they already know what the answer will be. (Better safe than sorry.) Because of this conservative attitude toward a questioning, it is unlikely that you will encounter all the worst tactics. We will start with some of the more forthright tactics before moving on to some methods that border on the unethical.

Tactic 1: Challenging Credibility

Challenging the credibility of a witness is one of the most common uses of cross-examination.[4] Questions may be raised to indicate that your perception (e.g., hearing) was faulty, your memory is inaccurate, your views are based on limited information, or your testimony is dishonest. Direct questions such as "Are you lying?" or "Did you really see that?" are unlikely. You are more likely to face indirect questions. For instance,

---

[4]For challenges to the credentials of expert witnesses, see Chapter 7.

"It's been over a year since you last spoke with Debra?" may be used to indicate your memory may not be so good after a year. There is nothing devious about this type of question. You can answer it honestly and allow people to draw their own conclusions. Similarly, if it was dark and you had difficulty seeing, then it was dark and you had difficulty seeing.

Consistency is key to whether your evidence will be believed. To impugn your credibility, the attorney could question exaggerations in your testimony, facts inadvertently or purposely omitted during the direct examination, or inconsistencies in your evidence. Were your direct examination to be perfect, it would include no exaggerations, omissions, or inconsistencies. However, testimony is rarely perfect, and you should avoid defensive responses. If you have committed one of these errors, keep your composure. Clarify your evidence in a "matter-of-fact" manner. "Yes, I did drive Paula home. I forgot to mention that in my original testimony." If there is a reason for an apparent inconsistency in your testimony, state the reason. "Perhaps I can explain the confusion. Philip acted intoxicated, but that was at our first session. At the second session, he acted sober."

Credibility can also be challenged by focusing on discrepancies between your evidence and that of another witness. State what you believe to be the truth. If you have a rational explanation for the discrepancy, then state it. "My observations may be different from Freida's because I started working with the family 3 months after they last saw Freida."

If your credibility is successfully impugned, the attorney who called you to the stand may undertake an effort to rehabilitate your evidence during the redirect phase of the examination . For instance, if the cross-examination has suggested that your memory has faded, she can ask you to refer to your notes to demonstrate that your oral testimony is consistent with what you wrote at the time of the event.

Tactic 2: Establishing Doubt

As noted in Chapter 1, different standards of proof are required in the various types of cases. In criminal trials, for example, the prosecution must prove its case "beyond a reasonable doubt." Accordingly, when an attorney is cross-examining for the defense, he may be trying to create just enough doubt to stave off a conviction. "Is it possible that someone other than Philip was responsible for Debra's injuries?" Well, anything is possible. Although you may agree that the attorney's proposition is "possible," you should also note how unlikely it is and your reasons for this.

In responding to attacks that attempt to establish doubt, be careful not to talk about the ultimate issue. In a criminal law case, clinicians are not responsible for deciding guilt or innocence. In fact, the language of the behavioral sciences does not include concepts such as guilt or innocence. Our language is the language of probabilities and relative likelihood. You may wish to talk about your estimate of the likelihood that an event may occur or the probability that an individual might engage in a specific act—but never talk about the guilt or innocence of a party.

Another way to reduce the impact of facts that the cross-examiner tries to use to impugn your testimony is to show that one set of facts may have multiple interpretations. The attorney may ask, "You said that Philip was perspiring and appeared drunk. Doesn't perspiration usually indicate that someone is hot?" You may offer a response that suggests a rival plausible hypothesis that may reasonably explain the observed behavior. Defend your interpretation with confidence, and do not respond defensively.

Tactic 3: Logic Funnel

When using a logic funnel, the attorney asks a series of questions intended to nudge the witness in a particular direction. By having the witness commit herself in earlier questions, she may be restricted in how she can answer later questions without contradicting herself (Cameron, 1995). "Is it normal practice in your agency to screen for suicidal ideation?" (Yes.) "So, you are supposed to screen in every case?" (Yes.) Then you should have screened in this case?" (Yes.) As you are being led down this funnel, answer honestly. If you are feeling squeezed toward the end of the funnel, take a few steps back: "I said that it was our standard practice to screen for suicidal ideation, and I would have done so in an ordinary case. This was no ordinary case, however, because . . . " Alternatively, you might recognize that you should have assessed for suicidal ideation and did not. Your response could be: "I should have performed such an assessment in this case. I did not perform that aspect of the assessment in this case." Such a response is honest, simple, and providing the needed information without becoming defensive.

Sometimes the logic in the line of questioning is only apparent on the surface. You may be able to distinguish your responses to different questions in the sequence without necessarily appearing to be inconsistent. This type of questioning may strike one as manipulative and may result in your feeling very cautious. Be on guard against feelings of anger or frustration during such questioning, and do not permit such feelings to adversely affect your testimony.

Tactic 4: Leading Questions

Leading questions suggest a particular answer to the respondent. They are used to encourage the witness to agree with the attorney's propositions. "From your opening testimony, it sounds as if you try to maintain very accurate case notes; wouldn't you agree?" Rather than confront you in a blatantly adversarial manner, the attorney is more likely to get positive responses with a friendly approach and by asking easy questions first. The attorney may present a series of "yes-able" questions that put the witness in the habit of agreeing. She may also ask a series of innocuous sounding questions to create a smooth sequence of questions and answers, lulling the witness into a false sense of security. To remain alert, consider each question independently. Take pauses. Change the speed and intonation of your voice.

Guard against the power of suggestion. If you do not agree with the attorney cross-examining you, say so. Some people who have a tendency to agree and avoid conflict must particularly pay heed. When you are asked a suggestive question, feel free to use your own words rather than accept the terms used by the questioning attorney. If an attorney asks you about "sexual abuse" and you respond with a comment about "sexual maltreatment," your choice of words might have significant implications. Consult with your attorney ahead of time about the type of language you should use, particularly with respect to legal terms. Also, if you are asked to describe something with a particular word and you disagree with the use of the word in the context of the question, do not use the word. Your testimony reflects your beliefs and opinions. Use terms that accurately reflect your ideas. Do not allow either attorney to mold your ideas to fit their theories. No one is more responsible for your choice of words, their intended meaning, and the effect they have on the court than you. Choose them wisely!

Finally, be attentive enough to correct questions based on faulty assumptions. Evelyn testified that Debra had nightmares, whereupon the attorney followed up with the question "Was Debra more likely to have nightmares about her father following a visit?" The attorney had effectively changed Evelyn's testimony by adding that the nightmares were about her father. Evelyn testified only that Debra had nightmares, but the follow-up question assumed that the nightmares were about her father. Evelyn should clarify this before responding about the frequency of the nightmares. She might say, "I testified that Debra had nightmares. I did not say that she had nightmares about her father. I did not say that she had nightmares upon returning from visits with her father. I apologize to the court if my testimony was unclear. My testimony is that Debra reported that she had nightmares."

Tactic 5: Feigned Ignorance

Attorneys sometimes present themselves as ignorant and ask naive questions. This behavior often puts the witness at ease, as thought the attorney had suddenly turned benign. The attorney may be fishing for evidence or trying to get the witness to open up. Remember to answer the questions concisely. Continue to respond in a respectful manner, even if the attorney's questions sound increasingly simple-minded or convey a sense of incompetence. Be aware that the attorney has not suddenly changed sides, and that she is likely to know much more than she is indicating through her chosen behavior.

Tactic 6: The Cutoff

Prepare for the possibility that your testimony will at some point be cut off by the attorney during cross-examination. Cutoffs are used to stop you from providing further information that is detrimental to the attorney's case. Remain polite. The tribunal or your attorney may intervene to provide you with an opportunity to complete your response. If necessary, ask the tribunal, "May I finish my answer, Your Honor?"

Tactic 7: Rapid Fire

In a tactic related to the cutoff, an attorney may ask questions in a machine-gun-like fashion. While this manner of questioning may simply be a way to speed up the process, it is more likely an attempt to get you to speak without having time to think about how to formulate your responses. Pace yourself deliberately. Frame each question clearly in your own mind, and answer each with due deliberation. Don't permit the opposing attorney to dictate the pace of your testimony.

In combination with rapid-fire questioning, some attorneys try to use intense eye contact with the witness. Intense eye contact makes it more difficult for some witnesses to slow down the pace and think. Remember that you can break intense eye contact by looking away. Looking up while you pause, for instance, demonstrates that you are thinking or trying to recall a visual memory. This will also break the spell that the lawyer is trying to place on you with the intense eye contact.

Saying something like "Let me think about my answer for a moment" takes control away from the attorney and places it squarely with you. If the attorney attempts to rush you, you might say something like "I am providing the best, most thorough answers to your questions so that I am most helpful to the court. Please, allow me to complete my answers."

This brings up the 5-second rule. It is a simple idea. During cross-examination, once you are asked a question, give the friendly attorney time to raise an objection before you begin to answer. Wait a moment and look over at the friendly attorney to see if she is preparing to object. If no objection is raised, then answer the question. If an objection is raised, do not offer any information until you are ordered to answer the question. You do not want to open the door on an area of inquiry that is outside the scope of your prepared testimony.

Tactic 8: Intentional Ambiguity

Intentional ambiguity is designed to confuse the witness and may get the witness to admit something that she did not intend. Ambiguity can be created through the use of language that has double meanings or through complicated questions. If Lori asked Sam, "Didn't you interview Paula and find that she was depressed?" then Sam would have to contend with two questions and one negative. Break complicated questions down into simple components and answer each question in sequence. "You have asked me two questions. The answer to the first is that I did interview Paula. The answer to the second question is that I am not an expert in diagnosing depression and did not report that Paula was depressed." Keeping your own statements simple helps to eliminate the possibility of being misunderstood.

Sometimes an attorney will make a speech rather than pose a question. Witnesses, not attorneys, are supposed to provide the evidence. If you do not hear a question in the attorney's comments, ask for the question to be clarified. When the attorney finishes his speech and looks to you for a response, you might say "I did not hear a question, Your Honor" or "I do not understand what you are asking of me."

Sometimes an ambiguous question is a "loaded question," meaning that the question attempts to discredit the witness by suggesting negative implications whether the witness agrees or disagrees. For example, the question "Isn't it true that psychologists have a long way to go before you can account for human behavior?" (Brodsky, 1991, p. 1) unfairly attempts to have the witness confess to a deficiency. The appropriate response to this type of question is to admit to the part that is true and then strongly rebut the part that is not true, as in, "This is a complex question that requires a complex answer. Yes, it is true that psychologists require further research to help explain many aspects of human behavior, but it is also true that there is strong research to support the premise that children like Debra are more likely to flourish when there is a lower level of conflict between divorcing parents."

The tribunal may frown upon such tactics as rapid-fire questioning and intentional ambiguity that are designed to confuse the witness. They detract from the purpose of the hearing, which is to get to the truth. If the tribunal does rebuke an attorney for such tactics, do not to take any pleasure in such a rebuke—at least not outwardly!

Tactic 9: Implying Impropriety

Some questions are designed to imply that you have done something dishonest, such as "Have you spoken to anyone about the answers you are giving today?" A witness may feel that, if they have discussed the case, then they may have breached some code of confidentiality or rule about evidence in court. If you have spoken to the attorney about your testimony before the trial, you should let the court know this. It is perfectly appropriate for a witness to discuss testimony ahead of time; the attorney may assist with "how" you present your information, but the substantive content should be what the witness knows about "the truth." In addition, you may have discussed the case with the client, your supervisor, and others; so what?

Another question that can throw you off guard is whether you are being paid to testify.[5] If you are working in an agency and going to court is part of your agency duties (as for a probation officer), admitting that you are being paid by the agency does not impeach your credibility. If you were hired to provide an assessment for the court, you should not be embarrassed to admit this fact (see "The Roles of Experts" in Chapter 7). However, it should be made clear that, although you are being paid to perform particular duties, you are not being paid to provide any particular testimony. You are being paid for your time to perform such duties, not for your testimony. A direct and nondefensive response is the best way to respond to a question that attacks your integrity.

Tactic 10: Rattling the Witness

There are a variety of ways to rattle a witness, most of which are of questionable ethics. Remember, however, that a good, tough question is not an unethical question. If a question is tough because it goes beyond your knowledge, you may have to admit that you do not know the answer. If the question is tough because you do not want to disclose harmful testimony, you may have to bite the bullet and provide the information requested: "Yes, I was present when my client was euthanized."

Ridicule, insults, sarcasm, and intimidation are questionable tactics. These techniques often backfire because the tribunal is inclined to disapprove of the attorney's tactics, resulting in a degree of sympathy for the witness. If an attorney antagonizes you, you will be less likely to cooperate with her questions. Also, the clinical and legal communities are small. If an attorney treats you poorly in one case, you may refuse to cooperate with her in the future. Still, some attorneys use these tactics and you might as well be prepared.

Intimidation can occur when the attorney uses close physical proximity, piercing eye contact, or a loud voice. If your space is being violated, feel free to move back if possible (remember, many witness chairs are bolted to the floor!). To avoid threatening eye contact, cast your eyes toward the tribunal or gallery (but not down, since this implies

---

[5]Brodsky (1991) suggests that forensic witnesses calculate their "objectivity quotient" by dividing the number of cases in which they agree with the hiring attorney by the total number of cases for which they are hired by an attorney to provide an expert opinion. If the quotient is high (e.g., over 75%) this may indicate a lack of objectivity. This statistic must be understood in context. For example, certain attorneys might prescreen for an expert who is known to agree with their position on the case.

you have something to hide). Do not try to match the attorney's volume nor try to speak over him. Maintain your composure. Try dropping the volume of your voice to deescalate the situation.

Try to remember to monitor yourself at all times when testifying. This includes monitoring your voice tone, loudness, and quality. Use the cognitive strategies discussed earlier, reminding yourself to keep calm and focused. Understand why the attorney might be trying to intimidate you; for example, he might be abrasive with all people or might have developed a false idea that attorneys have to be intimidating to carry out their role in an adversarial court hearing (Brodsky, 1991). Sit back and allow the attorney to rant and rage. You can counter with a calm, matter-of-fact response that shows that you remain in control of your testimony despite his theatrics.

Do not let ridicule or insults throw you off. Normally it is best to ignore them. You might feel that you want to say something like "Would you like to continue insulting me, or do you have questions that are relevant to the case?" However, it is usually best to allow the other attorney or the judge to respond to such inappropriate challenges during cross-examination. Avoid the temptation to enter the fray. Maintain your composure and focus on what you need to present to the court. Your attorney may step in to object or the tribunal may protect you from such tactics, regardless of whether anyone objects.[6] If a question is meant as an insult, you may ask the judge whether you have to answer it. Generally, leave objections to these types of questions to your attorney. Recall your techniques for dealing with anxiety and other feelings. Remind yourself that you are doing a good job and that you are trying to be helpful and honest. Focus on staying calm and in control.

Attacks on your personal life could involve questions about your sexual orientation, political affiliation or religion. In a divorce case, Evelyn might be asked if she were divorced and what happened in her marriage. Such questions are objectionable if they are irrelevant or intended primarily to intimidate or discredit you on inappropriate, prejudicial grounds.[7] You might ask the tribunal, "I am here in a professional

---

[6]If you do not have an attorney watching out for you during the proceedings, the tribunal is more likely to take active steps to protect you from abuse.

[7]In *Cheatham v. Rogers* (1992), the Texas Court of Appeals allowed examination related to the personal psychotherapy treatment of a court-ordered evaluator.

capacity. Can you help me with how I am supposed to reply to personal questions?" If the question is permitted, you are placed in a difficult situation. If you do not answer, you may be found in contempt of court or you may appear to be hiding something. You may decide to answer the question directly and matter-of-factly in order to minimize the impact of these questions and focus on the real issues of the case. You do not want to appear defensive. If inappropriate evidence is allowed into the hearing, this may create grounds for a subsequent appeal of the decision. Another strategy would be to preempt such attacks during the direct examination. Freida could disclose up front that she has a criminal record for possession of marijuana, or Sam could disclose that he had been reprimanded by his social work association 5 years ago for a breach of client confidentiality.

HEARINGS WITHOUT ATTORNEYS

Some legal processes are less formal and do not require the use of attorneys. The advantage in such a situation is that you have more control over your testimony. However, it also means that you need to prepare yourself and your evidence by selecting the relevant issues, determining the order of your presentation, and deciding on what to emphasize. The tribunal in such hearings may be more active and may even try to assist you with your testimony. The rules of procedure and evidence are likely to be less strict, providing you with greater latitude about what to say and when. Still, your evidence will have its greatest impact if it meets the tests of credibility described above.

It might be useful to obtain copies of the rules of evidence for such a hearing prior to attending. Review these evidentiary rules with your attorney and talk with colleagues who have attended similar proceedings.

TECHNOLOGY AND PROVIDING EVIDENCE

Traditionally, legal proceedings required live testimony with all participants present in a single hearing room. The use of technology is gaining greater acceptance in legal processes as a means of bringing people and evidence together more efficiently. Video and telephone conferencing allow people to retain the "live" part of the hearing, even though some of the participants are not in the same room. Audio and video recording of testimony have more limited use as they are past recordings and do not allow for cross-examination during the live part of the hearing. However, such recordings are used in selected circumstances (for example, to interview children in a less threatening environment than the hearing).

If you are going to provide testimony through one of these means, practice using the technology so that you can become accustomed to it and thereby present yourself more effectively. For instance, audiotapes and telephone conferences are limited to verbal testimony. Ensure that you are communicating clearly without the use of body language or other visuals (unless you have sent visuals such as pictures or graphs to the distant hearing location ahead of time). Even video technology is limited inasmuch as the focus of attention is determined by whoever is operating the camera rather than by people individually, who are free to focus their attention on anyone in the room. Consider the setup of the room where you are being recorded to ensure there are no distractions and to convey the sense of professionalism intended. While you want to be conscious of the microphone and camera, do not overplay to them. If you are recording your testimony to be played at a later date, try to use one continuous production. If you start and stop the recording, the decision makers may wonder what you have cut out.

Check to see whether there are any statutory provisions or case law precedents in your state about how to use such technology. These laws may address continuous versus discreet recordings and their admissibility. Further, these laws might differentiate between videotaping and audiotaping.

AFTER THE CROSS

After cross-examination, the attorney who conducted the direct examination can ask further questions to clarify your responses, clear up inconsistencies, or deal with other problems raised in the cross-examination. The attorney cannot raise new issues that should have been raised in the direct examination, nor can she ask leading or suggestive questions. Questions beyond the reexamination are rare. When you are dismissed from the stand, return to your previous seat in the hearing room. Remain there until the next break in the hearing.

When you are dismissed from the stand, it does not always mean that you are released to leave the courthouse. Only when you are told that you are dismissed and your testimony is no longer needed during the trial should you leave the courtroom.

When most witnesses leave the stand, they feel a sense of relief. Some feel dissatisfied. Others even report "posttestimony depression." You may feel you did not get a chance to tell your whole story, or that you could have done a better job—if only. . . . Some clinicians fantasize for days about what they could have said or what they wish they had been asked. Others feel that they spent too much time preparing, given the limited questions and cross-examination that actually occurred. Certainly, it is better to be over- rather than underprepared. If you were subjected to a personal attack, you may feel angry or embarrassed.

Debriefing is important. On legal issues, you may wish to consult with your attorney. For emotional issues, you may wish to debrief with another clinician. In unusual instances you may be recalled as a witness. Check with your attorney to see whether you need to avoid discussions until the case is over.

When you next meet with the attorney, you can discuss how well you presented your evidence and ask for tips on how to improve in the future. At a later date, you may even obtain a transcript of the hearing in order to review your performance.

Your attorney can help you interpret the results of the hearing. If Sam's evidence were to be challenged in a child protection hearing, it might seem as though the attorney was trying to make Sam appear incompetent. If the attorney succeeds, the court's decision about the child may not be as Sam had recommended. Still, the court cannot impose punishment on Sam (unless he has committed perjury). Instead, the court weighs the value of the evidence presented by Sam as having less importance than other, more relevant, evidence. While this type of experience is stressful, it is important to separate your best efforts from the results of the case decided by a decision maker whom you do not control.

Cases do not necessarily end at the conclusion of the hearing. Remember that, if a party is unhappy with the results of a hearing, there may be grounds for appeal (e.g., the tribunal was biased or certain procedures were not followed). In some cases an attorney may not even intend to win at trial; to establish a new precedent, cases must often progress to an appeal for a higher tribunal to make the decision. You may also undertake extralegal avenues of recourse, such as appealing to the government for changes in the law or participating in public policy formation.

Usually, at the end of "round 1," it just feels good to have your oral testimony over and done with.

Chapter 6

Clinical Records

Now that we have a picture of what happens at a hearing, let us take a step back to look at how to organize one's clinical practice in a way that best facilitates effective participation in legal processes. This chapter focuses on how to maintain clinical records that may end up being used in court or other adjudications.

Broadly defined, records include intake forms, confidentiality agreements, case progress notes, assessments, termination summaries, appointment books, statistics and research, psychological tests and inventories, pictures drawn by clients, photographs, billings, videotapes, correspondence and any other information stored by the clinician or agency. Sound record management practices are important because they:

- Enhance accountability.
- Facilitate supervision and case consultation.
- Help the clinician remember important case information when working with the client.
- Track the effectiveness of various interventions.
- Support a clinician's defense in a malpractice suit.
- Assist clinicians in preparation to be witnesses.
- Facilitate negotiation and settlement of legal cases.
- Provide documented evidence for legal actions.
- Satisfy legal requirements for regulated agencies and professionals.

Good records protect clients and the public as well as the clinician.[1] In clinical settings where every interaction or intervention has legal implications, clinicians may be required to adhere to different standards of record keeping. However, one cannot predict when a case may end up in legal proceedings, so "law-friendly" record keeping should be used universally. Each agency has unique recording requirements. In developing record-keeping policies, identify the most recent laws and codes of ethics relevant to your situation. Consult with an attorney when reviewing your agency's organization of records, the content of records, and client rights. Check also with your state association ethics or legal committee chairperson for current expectations within the state. Finally, some state and national associations publish a legal reference guide.

THE ORGANIZATION OF RECORDS

The organization of records includes how information will be gathered, entered into the system, preserved, and disposed of. Most agencies open a separate file for each client and maintain an ongoing record of all contacts. Note the type of contact in your notes: face-to-face, office meeting, home visit, telephone call, e-mail, or regular mail.

Consider whether you should create separate files for each member of a client family, for each member of a therapy group, or for different services for the same individual. When considering separate files for services provided to the same individual, consult your state's case law and ethical standards to ensure that such procedures are within the bounds of proper practice.

Freida prefers to use one file for a whole family or group because it is more efficient and enables her to describe systems information and group dynamics. However, if her file for the Carvey family is subpoenaed in a case involving Philip, she will have difficulty protecting Paula's confidentiality. Freida may be ethically compelled not to release information about Philip because such information contains information obtained from interviews with Paula. Without consent from both

---

[1] Consult your professional association for ethical standards and professional practice guidelines that pertain to record keeping. For cases involved in the legal process, record-keeping guidelines may require a higher level of clarity and organization that those recorded only for clinical purposes (CEGFP, 1991).

parties, the clinician may not be allowed to release information from a family session pertaining to only one person without violating the confidential relationship with others in the family for whom the therapist has no permission to release the information. One solution to such a quandary may be to provide a treatment summary that describes Philip's concerns while maintaining a confidential shield around information obtained from other people in the family session.

Another option is a hybrid approach. You could create a separate file containing sensitive or confidential information for each individual in a group or family, as well as a more general file for group or family processes.

Developing separate files for the same client may be appropriate in cases where some information is likely to be used in a legal proceeding but other information about the same client has less legal significance. For example, if Paula were to receive witness preparation support and vocational counseling from the same agency, separate files could be opened for each service. Information gathered by the witness preparation clinician may be subpoenaed. By opening a separate file for vocational work, this information may be protected from disclosure. A tribunal may allow certain sections of a file to be released while allowing other information unrelated to the case to remain undisclosed. However, the manner in which notes were originally recorded may make this approach impractical, particularly if the clinician interweaves facts about separate individuals and services in one case record.

Maintaining separate clinical files and releasing only those files that you as the therapist deem appropriate is a tricky issue. First, you need to be certain about the type of information requested by the subpoena. A *subpoena ducus tecum* requires that you provide all information about the client from all existing files. If the subpoena is less extensive in its breadth, then you may be allowed to provide limited information. Do not make a decision about what you can and cannot legally and ethically release without consulting an attorney as well as your state ethics code.

Generally, whoever gathers information should be responsible for entering the information into client records. This includes information obtained from both clients and collaterals (family members, employers, teachers, other clinicians, attorneys, etc.). Adjudicative processes give preference to firsthand information. If a receptionist gathers intake information, then the receptionist rather than the clinician should record this information with the receptionist's signature to acknowledge who recorded the note and when. If a clinician gathers information but has a secretary type her notes, then the clinician should review the typed notes to ensure that they are an accurate record. Notes should be signed by the person who gathered the information, warranting that the information is accurate. If the typed treatment notes are made for a case which you know may go to court, you may have a responsibility to maintain the dictated audiotape as well as the transcribed materials.

The timing of note taking can have great legal significance. Ideally, notes should be made contemporaneously with the events being recorded (i.e., during a session with a client, immediately following, or within 24 hours). Evidentiary rules assume that information recorded contemporaneously with the events is more likely to be accurate. Behavioral science research supports the fact that notes contemporaneously taken are more accurate than those recorded at a later time, even if it is later the same day. In a recent study, verbatim notes taken by highly trained interviewers were compared with the audiotaped versions of the interviews. The researchers found that even those interviewers with extensive training in *verbatim* note taking often got it wrong (Lamb et al., 2000). The moral of the story is that accurate recordings are critical. For legal purposes, it may be wise to record all your interviews electronically (Ceci & Bruck, 2000).

Record the date of the event as well as the date that the record was made and signed. If the notes were not made contemporaneously with an event, note the reason for this. Freida may not have entered her notes right away because she escorted Debra to the hospital on a medical emergency. If you follow a consistent practice of note recording, you can attest to your ordinary practice even if you do not have a distinct recollection of how a particular note was recorded. Be aware that notes recorded after an interview are likely to represent your general recollection of the session rather than your verbatim memory of specific statements. Therefore, when recording notes from a session after the fact, be careful not to indicate direct quotations since, as recent research has demonstrated, human beings are good at recalling the gist of a conversation but less accurate at recalling the precise language used (Bruck et al., 1999).

Organizing one's notes well may give them greater credibility. More than a few clinicians have been embarrassed during cross-examination by sloppy notes. Notes should be typed or handwritten in ink, in a consistent format. The use of Whiteout should be avoided because that could indicate that the records have been doctored. If you need to amend notes to add facts or to correct an inaccurate statement, identify clearly the date of the correction and the reason for the change.

Martindale (2000) recommends using notation paper that has numbered lines when taking notes that are to be used in court proceedings. He argues that the perception of organization adds to the court's perception of your credibility. For example, rather than saying that a note is referenced halfway down the page, using the Martindale method you could say, "The material to be reviewed is found on line 17 of page 6 of my notes." Now, *that* organizational scheme sounds impressive!

Records should be stored in a safe place to ensure confidentiality and to prevent tampering. If and when they are destroyed or disposed of, it should be done in a secure fashion, for example, through use of a shredder. The length of time that records should be kept may be specified by your funding source, by legislation, or by the code of ethics for your profession. Also, consider limitation periods for the types of actions that are more likely to arise from your practice. For example, civil law suits must generally be initiated within 6 years of the event that gave rise to the suit. For sexual assaults on children, actions may be started when the childhood memory is revived in adulthood. For serious criminal charges, there is no time limit. Consider whether the information in your files may be useful in potential actions, including a malpractice suit brought against you.

Storing information on computerized data systems permits its quick and efficient transfer. It also allows for compact storage of large quantities of information with easy retrieval. This technology can save time and enhance the presentation of your case if it goes to a hearing. However, technology also has pitfalls. Consider how to prevent tampering with information, computer viruses, lost data, and unauthorized access to client files. Both attorneys and computer programmers are struggling with how to ensure that stored data are safe and accurate. Use digital or hard copy backups as well as passwords and codes to protect sensitive information. Videotapes and audiotapes also require safe storage to prevent problems with unauthorized access and tampering. Finally, consider how to *permanently* erase information from disks or tapes; an unsuspecting clinician could easily forget that computers have "undelete" software that can restore data they thought they had destroyed.[2]

If you engage in communications via the Internet, be careful about what you say in your e-mails as well as how you send and store the messages. In spite of firewalls and password protections, it is possible for e-mail messages to be intercepted, either over the Internet or by hacking into someone's computer and stealing a password. Ensure that all written communications are fashioned in ways that anticipate their potential use in court under circumstances in which you would be asked to explain their meaning.

THE CONTENTS OF RECORDS

The perfect records for use in adjudication would be word-for-word transcriptions from audiotapes, sworn testimonials, and videotapes of all client interactions. However, since your primary role is as a therapist, these types of recording methods would prove overly burdensome in practice. Unless your primary role is to gather evidence as a potential witness, the contents of your records should be based primarily on what is clinically relevant and ethically required to provide competent clinical services. Because of our focus in this volume, the following section will highlight legal rather than clinical issues in discussing the contents of records.

Some agencies collect only information that is necessary to determine the appropriate service desired and to deliver the specific service being requested. This minimalist approach to record keeping is designed to protect client confidentiality in an environment where the evidence maintained can be illegitimately used to hurt or embarrass one's clients. In forensic contexts such as probation and child protection, clinicians have a specific role in documenting behavior that may later be cited in as evidentiary proceedings (Brown & Cox, 1998). When Sam investigates an allegation of child sexual abuse, he needs to document who is alleged to have assaulted whom, who is alleged to

---

[2]Consider using software specifically designed to permanently erase records. Also, check your hard drive or floppy disks for temporary files that contain confidential information. When disposing of a computer, the safest way to destroy all files is to reformat the hard drive.

have witnessed the assault, when it was alleged to have happened, where it was alleged to have taken place, and what the details of the alleged assault were (e.g., whether it was sexual and, if so, where the victim was touched and how; whether weapons were used; whether the victim consented). The level of detail required for Sam's records may go beyond what is required for therapeutic purposes. To ensure that the appropriate information is gathered and recorded, Sam needs to know the legal requirements for a conviction in criminal court or for intervening in a child protection case (e.g., is a medical examination required to support a conviction?). The manner in which evidence is gathered is also critical. In particular, cases involving children have been challenged because the clinician asked leading questions and, as a result of poor interview techniques, adversely influenced the child's information (Ceci & Bruck, 1993, 1995; Orbach & Lamb, 2001, Poole & Lamb, 1998; Sternberg, Lamb, Orbach, Esplin, & Mitchell, 2001). Clinicians who work as forensic experts require special training and knowledge (see Chapter 7).

Whatever the job related context, clinicians should keep concise records and follow a consistent system for collecting information. If certain information is deliberately omitted from a record, consider stating the reasons for doing so on the record and be prepared to defend your reasoning to an examining attorney, if need be. During mediation, Philip and Paula may discuss past marital infidelities but may ask Michael not to record them. Michael could note that historical information about the marriage was omitted at the request of the clients. If you use codes or shorthand, follow a key that explains these notations, use the codes consistently, and include the key in your records. Some professional practice guidelines (CEGFP, 1991) specifically warn against the use of codes or shorthand that cannot be understood by others reviewing your notes.

Contents of Progress Notes

The basic information to include for each progress note is:

- Who was involved in the contact
- What was the purpose for the contact
- The date, time, and location of the meeting

- What was the referral question
- Assessment information as described by each participant in the session
- Diagnosis, if any
- Summary of the diagnostic interview (including the usual and customary areas of exploration during the first session; e.g., suicidal or homicidal assessment, mental status)
- The basis for treatment decisions (including decisions not to treat)
- Treatment plan
- Possible legal involvement
- Any ethical issues raised and how they were handled

For example, if a client indicates suicidal or homicidal ideation—thoughts about harming herself or others—document this information and how you responded (e.g., whether you conducted a risk assessment, devised and had the client agree to a safety plan, referred the client for a second-level assessment, had the client dispose of drugs or a weapon, or warned a potential victim). Ensure that you also document issues such as child abuse, where there is a legal obligation to report (Kalichman, 2000). In using client statements as evidence in a proceeding, direct quotations have greater weight than paraphrasals. If you are unsure about the truth or basis of a client statement, include some details in your notes: "Paula appeared angry when she said she wanted to 'do Philip in' but indicated upon extensive interviewing that she had no plan or intention of carrying out any harmful acts." If the clinician wanted to protect Paula further, she could simply state, "Paula expressed anger because of Philip's threats," omitting any reference to Paula's own threats.

Since adjudications base decisions on facts (especially direct observations), speculation and secondhand information contained in client records may be of little use. For clinical reasons, it is important to record opinions and assessments. State these as opinions or assessments rather than as facts: "A possible interpretation for Debra's nightmares is . . . " Including the observations underlying your assessments and impressions can be useful clinically as well as in adjudication: "Debra disclosed that she continued to have nightmares about . . . " By noting the source of your information, you and others can reexamine your impressions at a later date to see if they are supported by other information brought to trial.

Secondhand information is often used for clinical assessments even though it may be considered unreliable in legal cases. For example, Sam might gather information on Debra from her teacher and physician. If secondhand information is useful to you for clinical purposes, include it in your records, but note the source of the information.

As with oral testimony, your records will have greater credibility if the information is free of bias and jargon. Some agencies, such as child protection services, have a specific obligation to maintain "full, fair, and balanced records." For example, Sam should include both positive and negative aspects of Philip's parenting relationship with Debra. While judgmental and bigoted language should be avoided in all cases, not all clinicians have a legal obligation to maintain balanced records. Freida's theoretical perspective focuses on client strengths. Her records will reflect this, deemphasizing client weaknesses. Other clinicians may omit damaging information about a client in order to protect the client, should a legal action arise. Although making such omissions may be legally permissible, consider whether it is clinically wise. (Note the discussion on thwarting disclosure, below.)

Be careful about making comments—written or verbal—concerning third parties. Such statements may increase the risk that your files will be subpoenaed by the third party about whom you allegedly made comments. This may damage your client's right to privacy. Further, you may be challenged for going beyond your authority, since the third party is not your client.

CLIENTS' RIGHTS

Clients should be aware of what will be kept in their records and what will not be kept, the policies for disposal, and provisions for gaining access to their records. Your agency should have procedures for clients to contest, correct, or revise the contents of their records, as well as policies to ensure that clients are aware of their rights.

All issues pertaining to confidentiality and disclosure should be documented in the client's records. Ideally, you have entered into a written service agreement with your client at the outset of providing treatment, explaining the client's right to confidentiality and the exceptions to it (described in Chapter 3). Before disclosing information to other people or agencies, you have asked the client to sign a consent to release such information. If the consent to release information is provided only orally, due to practical considerations, be sure to document this in your case notes. Then, have your client sign the written document as soon as possible. Any documents released to another agency should include a proviso that the information not be re-released without written permission from the client.[3]

During the intake stage of work with a client, the client has not yet entered into a service agreement. Since issues regarding confidentiality have not been settled between the agency and the client, the agency should limit documentation at the intake stage. When Michael received a call from Paula for mediation services, he documented the names and telephone numbers of the parties as well as the general nature of the issues to be mediated. He did not accept any historical information about the Carveys' situation nor the positions of the parties, preferring to wait until the parties had agreed to mediation and provisions regarding confidentiality. By doing so, he avoided setting himself up to be called as a witness in case the Carveys did not go ahead with mediation.

Consider situations in which disclosure in a legal proceeding is more likely to arise (e.g., a clinician who works with incest survivors, where disclosure is delayed and the clinician plays a role in bringing a formal report to the police). Pay particular attention to the contents of the records and the extent to which certain information can be damaging to your client if a case proceeds to a hearing. If clients keep diaries or prepare artwork as part of your intervention, consider whether they should keep these records in their own possession. If these documents are not in your possession or control, then you do not have to submit them if your records are subpoenaed. However, the same documents could be subpoenaed from your client.

USING RECORDS AT A HEARING

Records may be brought into evidence at hearings in three ways. The first method, use of reference notes to help refresh the clinician's memory, was described in Chapter 5. In order to use notes to refresh your

---

[3]The provision not to re-release information without the client's written authorization may not apply when you release your case file to an investigator or evaluator who is preparing a report to the court. By definition, when documents are released to an investigator or evaluator for the court, the released information becomes part of the court's file and is available to be examined by the attorneys and the court.

memory, the notes must have been made contemporaneously with the events recorded, and you must have an active memory of the events at the time of the hearing.

The second method of bringing notes into a hearing arises when the witness has forgotten the events recorded. The notes may be entered into evidence as "past memory recorded." This type of evidence is not as persuasive as evidence provided when you use notes to refresh your memory. If you do not have a current recollection of the events, the contents of the notes cannot be challenged through cross-examination. Your notes may be unreliable as evidence, since they were developed for clinical purposes rather than for litigation. The information in clinical notes is often based on hearsay rather than sworn testimony and direct observations. Further, facts and opinions may be intermingled, and the information in your notes may be taken out of context. However, by following the guidelines suggested in this chapter, your notes are much more likely to withstand the legal tests of credibility even if you do not have a current recollection at the time of the hearing.

The third method of bringing client records into a hearing occurs when the person who took the notes is not available as a witness (e.g., if Freida left her agency and could not be located). Tribunals may admit clinicians' notes as "business records." Business records are documents created in the normal course of business and not in contemplation of a particular legal action. Business records are most often used for less contentious issues. If an issue is highly contentious, the tribunal may disallow use of the records because there is no opportunity to cross-examine the accuracy of the information nor the way in which the opinions were formulated. If you are planning to leave an agency or move to another location, consider leaving a forwarding address for clients or others who may need to call you as a witness. Your professional obligations may continue even after you have ended your working relationship with a client or agency. Unfortunately, most clinicians would rather not be called as a witness after they have moved on.

Videotapes can be very persuasive in court. They can provide accurate, objective, and complete recordings of what happened. In an investigation of allegations of child abuse, for example, a videotape of a child's interview with a clinician will help determine the quality of interviewing experienced by the child and may assist in teaching the judge either about the accuracy of the child's statements or how the child's statements may have been influenced by the investigator's techniques (Orbach & Lamb, 2001). Videotapes may also have an impact on the perception of witness credibility. Observing a child witness in a properly conducted interview may have a significantly more powerful effect on the judge and jury than the testimony of the clinician who interviewed the child. The decision makers can hear the child on a first-hand basis rather than having to rely on the clinician's interpretations of the interview. Videotaped interviews require specific expertise. Otherwise, their validity can easily be challenged on the basis of improper or leading questions (Ceci & Bruck, 1995; Poole & Lamb, 1998; Woodbury, 1996).

THWARTING DISCLOSURE

Clinicians often wish they could prevent disclosure of records. Some reasons are valid, others not. Clinicians treating victims of sexual assault, for example, are concerned that their clients will be subjected to intense scrutiny before and during the trial of the alleged perpetrator. Defense attorneys often seek complainants' records from clinicians, crisis services, and transition houses. Defense attorneys may use this information to try to challenge the credibility of the complainant. An attorney may try to discredit the complainant by saying that she is emotionally unstable, tends to fabricate stories, or is motivated to lie because she is trying to hide having had sex with someone else. Some laws have been enacted to limit interrogations of complainants. For instance, the so-called rape shield law restricts questions about the complainant's past sexual behavior. Still, attorneys are permitted to ask many types of questions that might embarrass or undermine the perceived credibility of the complainant. Defense attorneys may try to subpoena a clinician's records for evidence that the complainant consented to sex or that the complainant is an unreliable witness (e.g., due to false memories induced in therapy, disassociation, or other mental instability). In complaints of child sexual abuse, defense attorneys may try to gain access to records from the complainant's school or group home clinicians. These records may contain a history of dysfunction, emotional problems, and acting out behavior. If a clinician wants to protect his client from disclosure of this type of information in a public legal process, virtually every option has its drawbacks. Before adopting any of these options, consult with your attorney, professional association, or other expert on law and professional ethics.

Minimal Records

To protect their clients, some clinicians resort to maintaining minimal records (e.g., limiting details to the name of the client, the problem presented, and the dates seen). They deliberately exclude any information that could harm the credibility of the complainant or embarrass her. Unfortunately, some of this information may be clinically important, legally relevant, and ethically necessary. Suicidal or homicidal thoughts, alcohol or drug use, and high levels of stress are just a few examples. Although minimal records may thwart disclosure in legal processes, they may not meet the standards required for competent clinical practice. Further, the clinician can still be called to testify about client information not included in case records.

Double Records

Some clinicians keep two sets of records—an official set and a personal set. The official set excludes potentially damaging information. The personal set includes all information, assessments, and speculations that the clinician uses for her own purposes. Although some clinicians believe that a subpoena applies only to the official records, all records are subject to subpoena. Some clinicians hide the fact that they have a set of unofficial records. However, if found out, that failure to disclose all records can result in charges against the clinician. The question raised by some clinicians is "How will anyone know?" The real question is "What does your sense of ethics and risk taking tell you?" Few agencies or professional associations would officially condone hiding a second set of records. There is no ethical foundation for keeping two sets of records. Ethically as well as statutorily, one set of records is what is appropriate.

Coded Information

Some clinicians use secret coding to make parts of their records indecipherable to people unfamiliar with the coding. Some codes are so subtle that the reader does not even know that coding is being used (e.g., a double asterisk may denote past suicide attempts). During a hearing you may be asked to explain your codes or shorthand. If it appears that you have deliberately tried to mislead the reader, your credibility as a witness may be called into question. Further, if someone else in your agency needs to refer to your records, will she be able to understand what you have written?

As indicated earlier, if you know in advance that your case may be involved in a legal proceeding, you may have an ethical obligation to maintain clear notes without the use of code or shorthand, so that other people reviewing your work, now or at a later time, can understand the meaning of your records.

Doctoring or Disposing of Documents

If there is no impending legal process, clinicians are free to amend their records. In many agencies, supervisors or agency attorneys periodically review case records and suggest changes to avoid future problems (e.g., to remove judgmental language, bias, or speculation). Clinicians are also free to dispose of records, within the policies of the agency and the standards of the profession. Michael's mediation association, for example, suggests that mediators maintain records for at least 6 months after mediation has been terminated. However, if a clinician is aware of an impending legal process or has been subpoenaed, doctoring or destroying documents can result in such charges as contempt of court or obstruction of justice, malpractice suits, and professional disciplinary actions. Once again, the question may arise, "How will anyone know?" Before shredding your files, you might want to explore the frequency with which fraudulently motivated shredding has been unearthed and exposed.[4]

Even if you have no records, you can still be called as a witness. You may have limited value as a witness, particularly if you have no current recollection of the events in question. However, keeping records might actually help your client, since premature disposal of records can hurt your credibility as a witness. Finally, a clinician without records may be more vulnerable to malpractice suits (e.g., where a client later

---

[4]In one case where a social worker shredded records of a meeting with a sexual assault complainant, the court stayed the proceedings against the man accused of the sexual assault. The court found that, because the accused was denied access to the documents, his right to a fair trial (including full answer and defense) was breached (*Regina v. Carosella*, 1997).

alleges that the clinician induced a false memory of abuse) or complaints before a licensing board for failure to comply with ethical standards of record keeping.

Lying

As noted throughout this volume, when clinicians are involved in legal processes they are expected to tell the truth. Depending on their priority of values, some clinicians may be tempted to intentionally lie to protect clients or themselves. Freida believes her records will embarrass Paula, so Freida considers telling Lori that she has already destroyed them. Sam does not want to be called as a witness, so he wonders whether to tell the court he has no current recollection of any of his notes (a convenient memory lapse). These types of tactics can thwart disclosure. However, you risk charges of perjury and professional misconduct, as well as a negative perception for both you and your profession. Professional organizations, agencies, and judges will rarely condone lying, even if the witness honestly believes she has good intentions.[5]

Given the foregoing dilemmas, how does a clinician balance these risks and conflicting interests? If a significant part of your mandate is to collect evidence, then this takes precedence in the way that you gather and store information. If your primary role is that of a helping professional, then your records should be designed primarily to meet your needs as a clinician. Bear in mind the potential legal pitfalls. In many fields of practice there are few conflicts between the clinical and legal requirements for proper record keeping. In areas where conflicts arise, there may be no ideal solution.

---

[5]The types of rare examples include necessity (e.g., lying in order to prevent a person from being killed when there is no other alternative) or to escape pernicious treatment by a rogue state (e.g., Jews and other persecuted people who lied to escape Nazi Germany).

Chapter 7

Expert Witnesses

Up to this point, we have primarily been discussing fact witnesses. This chapter focuses on expert witnesses. Whereas a fact witness provides testimony about direct knowledge of facts at issue in a legal proceeding, a person who qualifies as an expert witness can provide opinions as well as fact evidence. Court proceedings tend to be strict about limiting opinion evidence to recognized experts. Other types of hearings may allow people to express opinions without necessarily requiring that the person be legally qualified as an expert.

The rationale for restricting most witnesses to direct observations relates to the division of roles in an adjudicative process. The role of a witness is to state her knowledge of the relevant facts. The role of the judge or other decision maker is to determine the truth, based on a hearing of all of the witnesses. To come to a determination, the decision maker needs to formulate opinions. If a witness was permitted to state opinions during the hearing, he could usurp the role of the decision maker. An exception is made for people who qualify as experts, because experts can assist the decision maker by virtue of their specialized knowledge and experience. To some clinicians, these distinctions sound unduly rigid. However, if you wish to play the game, you need to know the rules.

Clinicians come from a range of disciplines that allow them to assist tribunals through their expertise. Social workers might be called upon to deliver assessments of individuals in relation to their families and other systems in their social environments. Among the more commonly used experts in court are clinicians who specialize in forensic mental health issues such as forensic psychology, forensic psychiatry, and forensic social work. They may be expert in criminology, child development, human motivation, mental illness, or family violence. Psychiatrists and psychologists are frequently called in legal proceedings to provide an assessment of an individual's mental condition (e.g., competence to stand trial or existence of mental disorders that render the individual not responsible for his actions). Psychiatrists might render medical opinions, while psychologists might offer opinions about psychological test data. Just because a clinician is recognized by her peers as an expert does not mean that the clinician will be qualified as an expert in a legal proceeding. The clinician may be called as a fact witness, in spite of her expertise. The fact that you are not called as an expert in a particular case should not be taken as a slight against your competence.

The following sections describe the various roles of experts, the admission of expert evidence, and the ways in which an expert may be selected for a particular case. In the latter sections of this chapter, we revisit the direct examination and cross-examination, with a focus on expert witnesses. Finally, we explore the issues of reliability and validity of expert testimony in reference to clinical knowledge and research.

THE ROLES OF EXPERTS

A clinician who specializes in gathering, preparing, or presenting information for legal processes is called a forensic expert.[1] Clinicians can play a variety of forensic roles, including Hired Gun, Advocate, Impartial Expert, Consultant, and Ivory Tower Academic (Wasyliw, Cavanaugh, & Rogers, 1985). In some of these roles, the clinician is not called as a witness but rather is used behind the scenes to assist a party in strategizing or preparing for a legal proceeding. This is sometimes referred to as a "nontestimonial" role and may be specified in advance in a letter of engagement from the attorney who hires you.

---

[1]Forensic experts require very specific training and experience. Because forensic work is so specialized, we would not be able to do justice to any particular field without writing a separate book on that field (e.g., Ben-Porath, Graham, Hall, Hirschman, & Zaragoza, 1995; McCann & Dyer, 1996; Morgan, 1995; Myers, 1998). If you plan to act as a forensic expert, this book provides a good foundation, but you need to proceed beyond this base.

In some cases clinicians play two or more of these roles. When assuming more than one role, you must be careful not to engage in unethical behavior. For example, if you have been a client's therapist, it is unwise to perform an evaluation for the courts; it is not only unethical to do so but also tends to undermine your objectivity and thus the usefulness of information brought before the court.

Hired Gun

The Hired Gun is an expert hired by one party. In spite of the general perception that a hired gun is paid to support a particular finding or position, the ethical responsibility of any forensic specialist is to serve the best interests of the court. The best interests of the court are served when the expert witness performs in an objective, impartial manner regardless of who hires him. Unfortunately, there are still some experts who sell their services to the highest bidder or will testify for the people who hired them rather than testifying for the truth. However, more often than not, a forensic specialist hired by one side will provide an honest appraisal of the facts and, if permitted to testify, will provide an honest accounting of the accumulated data and its derived interpretations.

In the past it would not have been unusual in a custody battle such as the Carveys' dispute for Philip to hire a family and divorce specialist to rebut Evelyn's assessment that Debra's best interests would be served by an order for sole custody with Paula. According to the Hired Gun's assessment, Philip should have custody of Debra. Although the Hired Gun met with Philip, he did not meet with Paula in arriving at his assessment.

Since the 1990s, judges, attorneys, and clinicians have increasingly become aware that it is unethical to offer an opinion about custody or visitation access without having evaluated the entire family system (American Psychological Association, 1995). In today's climate, Philip's expert would likely be challenged by the opposing attorney, citing statements in various codes of ethics and professional practice guidelines as well as published texts in the field of custody evaluation. Thus, a Hired Gun's assessment that offers predictable opinions about custodial placement is likely to be given little weight by the judge nowadays. And, if the judge understands current forensic mental health practice, the Hired Gun's testimony may negatively affect the judge's perception of the expert's credibility.

Unfortunately, the practice of seeking out predisposed Hired Guns to support one's case continues. From an ethical perspective, it is important to remember that, no matter who hires you, your responsibility is to the truth of your work and its accurate and honest representation in a court of law.

In a different example, a Hired Gun could be a published expert who strongly believes in a particular position and is willing and able to talk about that perspective in court. The Specialty Guidelines for Forensic Psychologists (CEGFP, 1991) specifically suggest that the role of a forensic specialist is to be committed to fairness and justice in the legal system. This mission can be accomplished only by the honest exchange of ideas that are then critically evaluated by the judge or jury. Presenting only one side without even referring to alternative perspectives misleads the court into believing there is only one side to the argument. For example, if Freida were to have a malpractice suit filed against her, she might decide to hire an expert who supports the use of her unorthodox methods of intervention. This expert might also be able to testify that there are research studies, clinical literature,[2] and local community standards that support the use of such methods.

Advocate

The Advocate supports a certain position based on allegiance to a particular philosophy, affiliation, belief system or set of values. For example, the Hired Gun described above might be known to favor joint custody. He would advocate for joint custody in Philip's case, notwithstanding the allegations of abuse. Advocates are used extensively in hearings involving public policy issues (e.g., euthanasia or the rights of disadvantaged groups). Advocates may be paid to act as witnesses but are sometimes willing to testify without pay because they believe that testifying will advance their cause.

Within forensic literature some argue that a forensic specialist should never take on the role of advocate (Gould, 1998). From an ethics perspective, forensic specialists have an obligation to the court to present rival, plausible alternative hypotheses that might explain a set

---

[2]See Shuman and Sales (1998) for an excellent discussion of different admissibility standards to be applied to clinical and empirically based research.

of data. If an advocacy position means presenting only the arguments for a particular view, then this would be unethical.

Impartial Expert

The Impartial Expert is hired to provide an independent evaluation of a case. He reviews all data—pro and con—and forms an opinion on the basis of the data rather than simply putting forward the desired position of the side that is soliciting his services. An example of an impartial expert is an independent mental health professional appointed by the court to answer specific psycholegal questions for which the court needs an expert's opinion.[3] In the Carvey situation, Evelyn is also an impartial expert, as she was hired by both parties to provide a psychosocial assessment.[4] For a sample of an Informed Consent Form that explains the role of an Impartial Expert, see Appendix C. Also, see Appendix D for a sample of an Initial Letter to Attorneys after an Appointment Order.

Ivory Tower Academic

The Ivory Tower Academic is an expert in a particular field of science who does not have any connection with or knowledge about the specific facts of the case. In an inquest into a suicide case, an Ivory Tower Academic could be called to testify about the incidence of suicide among people in certain treatment populations (e.g., alcohol abusers). She may also comment about the relevance of scientific inquiry or about public policy issues (e.g., the need for preventive services).

A more positive term that has been used to describe this role is "educator to the court." Rules of evidence support the use of an expert to teach the court about areas of knowledge that are "outside the keen awareness of the average layman." The role of the educator to

---

[3]See Amundson, Daya, and Gill (2000) and Gould (1999a, 1999b) for more details about the importance of clearly defining the psycholegal questions to be considered in a child custody evaluation.

[4]There is recent case law from the Vermont Supreme Court that an impartial expert hired by the parents rather than appointed by the court is not covered under immunity statutes and therefore could be subject to legal action (*Politi v. Tyler*, 2000).

the court is best served by providing reliable and relevant information about a particular area of behavioral science research. If the expert is able to relate the research findings directly to specific fact patterns in the case before the court, the information may be judged to be helpful to the court.[5]

In some instances when you are hired as a educator to the court by one side in a legal dispute, the hiring attorney will scrupulously not talk directly with you, not provide you with specific information about the case, and not help you to prepare your testimony. Here, the attorney's aim is to preserve for the court the perception that you are free of bias about this particular case. If your role is to provide information drawn only from the research or clinical literature, then there may be no need for you to know anything about the case before the bench. If this approach is effectively implemented, the court will view your testimony as more objective than if you had been briefed on the facts of the case or had prematurely formed impressions about which side should prevail.

Consultant

The Consultant is hired by one party to assist the attorney with preparation and development of a case. The Consultant may or may not be used to testify as a witness. The functions of the Consultant may include:

- Identifying issues, collecting evidence, and building the case (e.g., compiling diagnoses and reports from other clinicians).
- Evaluating evidence (e.g., reviewing the process used for psychological testing; critiquing the credibility of information provided by other expert witnesses who may be called to testify; evaluating the validity and reliability of research in the area).
- Assisting an attorney in determining whether a reasonable cause of action exists (e.g., whether Michael breached his ethical obligation regarding confidentiality).

---

[5]See Krauss and Sales (1999) for a discussion of the legal concepts of reliability, relevance, and helpfulness as applied to expert testimony in the behavioral sciences.

- Identifying and evaluating negative factors in the case (e.g., what evidence goes against Philip's claim for custody and access).
- Preparing a technical report explaining clinical concepts in terms that can be understood by the attorney.
- Preparing questions to ask expert witnesses at the hearing for examination of friendly witnesses and cross-examination of opposing witnesses.
- Evaluating or interpreting expert evidence adduced during the hearing.
- Developing diagrams for presentation at the hearing (e.g., genograms to depict family relationships; charts that illustrate research findings).
- Identifying precedent cases involving expert evidence.
- Advising about the selection of jurors (e.g., what types of questions to ask prospective jurors; what types of verbal and nonverbal cues to look for; how to interpret various responses, attitudes, or values).

For a sample of a Service Agreement for an Expert Witness hired in a Consultant's role, see Appendix A.

Although there is potential for abuse in each of the five roles, those experts who are engaged as Advocates and Hired Guns are most susceptible to questions about their motivations, ethics, and practices. For most adjudications, the ideal expert witness takes an objective stance and serves as an impartial educator. If an expert is hired by one party to provide evidence, the expert may experience covert and overt pressure to distort data to support an opinion or to select information supportive of a particular position. Ethical obligations require professional clinicians to act honestly, making sure they do not misrepresent available research or professional knowledge. A clinician who sees herself as an advocate needs to be careful about how she presents herself—so as not to taint her credibility in a particular case or her reputation more generally (e.g., if she always provides the same type of recommendation, regardless of the specifics of a case).

Consider a case in which a psychologist is hired to provide testimony concerning the accuracy of an eyewitness account. A psychologist who sees herself as an Advocate might emphasize those memory and perceptual factors that suggest inaccuracy, such as the briefness of the exposure or the likely stress experienced by the eyewitness. A psychologist who takes on the role of an Impartial Expert will discuss factors that affect eyewitness performance, including lighting conditions or a short retention interval (McCloskey, Egeth, & McKenna, 1986). Impartiality and the perception of impartiality are vital to the expert witness's credibility. In public policy or legislative proceedings, advocacy for a particular point of view is more acceptable. Still, the advocate will probably be viewed as more credible if she bases her position on objective facts or research rather than on emotional or ideological appeals.

ADMITTING EXPERT EVIDENCE

For expert evidence to be admitted into a court hearing, the evidence must be relevant, necessary, and delivered by a properly qualified expert. The evidence must also meet other rules of admissibility (or inadmissibility, such as exclusionary rules based on public policy). As noted earlier, other tribunals will generally admit expert evidence without such strict guidelines for exclusion. However, the weight given to the evidence may be related to similar factors.

As with other forms of evidence, expert evidence must be directly relevant to the issues in the case. For clinicians, this means that you must know how your expertise and opinions relate to the legal issues at stake. It is no use giving your opinion that Philip was at fault for the breakup of the marriage if legally this has no relevance to how the issue of custody is determined. By understanding the legal issues, you will be better able to focus your testimony on the key issues.

The rule that expert evidence must be "necessary" limits the expert to providing opinions or recommendations that are beyond the expertise of the decision makers. Is there knowledge, skill, or information that a layperson does not have but would require in order to formulate an opinion or conclusion? If the area of knowledge is within the grasp of decision makers, then there is no need for an expert to provide the information. For example, common sense tells us that if a person purchases a gun one day and the very next morning he puts on a mask and shoots his wife while she is sleeping, the murder is likely premeditated. An expert would not be needed to draw this conclusion. Alternatively, an expert's opinion may be useful concerning the chances that a given defendant might repeat offensive behavior. One of the most common uses of clinicians as experts is to provide clinical diagnoses or assessments for such things as mental disorders, drug dependencies, or instances of family dysfunction.[6]

Another role for an expert is to explain theories and scientific information. But what if a court has been educated about a particular theory in prior cases? The concept of "judicial notice" is a legal principle that allows courts to admit a specific scientific theory or finding that is so well established that it is common knowledge and does not require independent proof of its truth at the hearing. Battered child syndrome was once a highly debated issue in certain courts. Its existence has now been so firmly established by expert witnesses that some courts take judicial notice of it. If the court takes judicial notice of certain information, it is no longer necessary to call an expert witness on the matter.

To be "qualified" as an expert, the witness must have a defined knowledge or skill in the area related to the opinion evidence that the expert intends to provide. A clinician may qualify as an expert in relation to some issues but not others. If Sam were admitted only as an expert in child development and the impact of sexual abuse on children, for example, he would not be permitted to provide opinions about Philip's propensity to commit acts of physical abuse against his wife. Assessments for people from a particular cultural group may require specific training, knowledge, and experience with that group (Gothard, 1989b). An expert with competence in ethnospecific practice can provide important services to tribunals as cultural interpreters. As a qualifying expert, your testimony is limited to the areas for which you have been admitted as an expert. If there are several areas that require your testimony, seek to be qualified as an expert in each area of your potential testimony.

There is no single test for who may qualify as an expert. The court will generally consider the witness's training, experience, and knowledge, as well as her ability to use judgment in a particular field of science. Historically, courts have been more likely to recognize clinicians as experts if they came from medicine or other legislatively recognized professions.[7] If a clinician is licensed or accredited by a professional

---

[6]Within a forensic context, performing the assessment of a mental disorder may require forensic rather than clinical methods and techniques.

[7]Psychiatry is still often treated as the mental health profession with the highest status. Tribunals often defer to the opinions of psychiatrists. This may be particularly discouraging to a clinician who has more specialized experience or greater research support than the psychiatrist.

body, the court is assured that the clinician meets the standards for knowledge, skill, experience and education required by that body. However, being a member of a professional association does not guarantee qualification as an expert, and many clinicians who are not regulated professionals can still qualify as experts. If you do not qualify as an expert, you may still be able to provide fact evidence that can be used to support the opinions of other experts. For example, Sam could report his observations of Philip's behavior, and a university-affiliated criminologist could interpret this behavior.

If you are going to be called to testify as an expert witness, a current *curriculum vitae* (c.v.) or professional résumé is essential. The information in your c.v. should be well organized, accurate, and complete. Because decision makers are provided with a copy that they take away, the c.v. carries a lasting impression. Do not inflate your credentials, since the c.v. is subject to cross-examination. Your c.v. should include the elements listed in the accompanying Box.

Elements of a *Curriculum Vitae*

- Your professional title
- Contact information
- Training and education
- Degrees and professional licenses
- Years of experience
- Employment history
- Supervisory experience
- Special awards or citations
- Provision of training
- Prior court experience (issues, representing which side, level of court, whether qualified as an expert; county and state in which you were qualified)
- Work under recognized experts
- Memberships in professional organizations

- Books or articles written
- Positive book reviews or judicial comments on your work
- Professional speaking experiences
- Ongoing supervision or case consultation
- Professional development and continuing education courses you have taken
- Consultation work
- Code(s) of ethics to which you prescribe
- Methods of practice to which you prescribe
- Professional development and continuing education courses you have taught
- Recognized specializations

Gear your c.v. to the specific areas of expertise required for the types of opinions you will be providing. If Lori calls a therapist to testify about Philip's competence to stand trial, the therapist could highlight her most relevant credentials by including brief (or expanded) explanations of them. If your c.v. looks interesting, people are more likely to spend time reading it.

In terms of the process at the hearing, the attorney calling you informs the tribunal that he intends to qualify you as an expert. Sometimes the other party will not contest the witness's expertise, and the process of qualification is straightforward. The attorney will take you through your c.v. and highlight areas most relevant to the opinions to be given. Your attorney can also deal with weaknesses in your background. Michael may have authored few articles or books, but this can be explained largely by the overwhelming time demands associated with his extensive hands-on experience and study in mediation.

You may be asked an open-ended question about your education and experience, in which case you should be prepared to summarize your background in an organized and detailed manner. The other attorneys can cross-examine you on your qualifications. The judge has the responsibility for ruling on whether you qualify as an expert who can express opinion evidence. Even if the opposing attorney admits you as an expert witness, your attorney may still take you through your qualifications in significant detail to ensure that your evidence will be given due weight. Your attorney can also lay a foundation for your expertise in particular areas, since the opposing attorney may try to narrow the range of your expertise (Chisholm & McNaughton, 1990). Having the attorney walk you through your c.v. also provides you with some time to get comfortable on the witness stand while you engage in discussing a topic that requires little pressure. No matter how often you testify, take the time to review your credentials in some detail so that you can settle into the witness chair and become comfortable with the surroundings.

The manner of your presentation may be more important than your actual list of credentials. This is a time to be neither too humble nor too egotistical. A problem facing social workers, in particular, is that the profession and many agencies promote generalist practice. For example, Sam's child protection agency encourages its workers to be familiar with a broad range of child welfare issues rather than to pursue specialization in incest, neglect, and the like. While a generalist background may be useful for clinical purposes, lack of specialization makes it difficult for Sam to ever qualify as an expert witness. Client-centered clinicians face a similar dilemma. Since they view clients as experts in their own lives, client-centered clinicians often find it difficult or distasteful to provide diagnoses or "expert" recommendations for their clients. This view may limit such clinicians to providing factual evidence.

While some clinicians shy away from being considered as experts, others may want to enhance their ability to act as expert witnesses. By the time you are called to participate in a particular case, it may be too late. If you want to qualify as an expert, ensure that you obtain the requisite education, experience, and certification. These credentials enable you to demonstrate that you have acquired the appropriate knowledge and skills for competence in your field. Research, professional presentations, and publications will add to your credibility. Strive for consistency in what you say or publish, as inconsistencies can undermine your perceived trustworthiness. Keep your knowledge up to date by reading journals or attending seminars and conferences. Working with recognized experts can enhance your reputation. Developing positive relationships with colleagues in your field of practice is also important, since they may be called upon to evaluate your competence as a clinician and as an expert witness.

Although expert evidence must meet the primary criteria for admissibility—that is, be reliable, relevant, and helpful—expert evidence can also be excluded on grounds of inadmissibility, including:

- If the probative value of the evidence is outweighed by its prejudicial effect.
- If the time necessary to present the evidence is incommensurate with its value.
- If the effect on the adjudicator is out of proportion to its reliability.

The main fear with expert evidence is that the fact finder will be unduly influenced by an expert witness. Consider if Sam were to provide evidence, based on his assessment, about the possible risk of violence associated with Philip's current behavior. It is difficult to predict risk of violence with a high degree of certainty; yet, a judge or jury may be tempted to believe that Philip poses a high risk to Debra's safety—even if this is not the evidence that was presented. Sam's task is to educate the court about how Philip's risk factors may or may not present a danger specifically to Debra, including the relative reliability of the expert opinions being offered.

Tribunals often place a great deal of faith in the opinions of expert witnesses. A clinician can spend much more time than the tribunal studying and assessing an individual. The clinician is also respected for his special expertise. To illustrate the difference between how tribunals treat expert evidence and evidence from laypersons, consider the use of professionally prepared presentence reports versus victim impact statements. Victim advocates have argued that criminal courts give little weight to victim impact statements when sentencing. Often, the court will simply follow the report of the expert who wrote the presentence report. The statement drafted by the victim may be emotionally charged, use biased language, and be written with poor grammar and spelling. The presentence report is balanced, well written, and uses language that speaks to the concerns of the judge. If a clinician wants the victim's perspective to be given weight, the clinician needs to include this in the presentence report.

Another rule of evidence, the ultimate issue doctrine, suggests that experts are not allowed to provide opinions about the ultimate issue in dispute (e.g., Federal Rules of Evidence, Rule 704). Under this doctrine, if Freida were sued for malpractice, another clinician would not be permitted to testify directly that Freida's interventions constituted malpractice. The court is responsible for drawing the ultimate conclusions in a case, not the witness. An expert witness is only supposed to educate the tribunal. Courts are now allowing experts to provide evidence closely related to the ultimate issue; however, they are strictly applying the rules of relevance and necessity. If the court is just as capable as the expert in drawing a conclusion, then the expert is permitted to provide facts or knowledge, while the court retains the responsibility for drawing the ultimate conclusion.

Be careful about situations where an attorney may entice you into saying things that you are not authorized to say or have no foundation to say. Recently Jon was involved in a case in which a clinician provided a sworn affidavit to the court stating that her client was clearly innocent of all charges against him. During trial, when the attorney asked her to show where she found the diagnostic category of "innocent" in the DSM, the clinician realized that she had offered a legal rather than a mental health opinion. Once written and then testified to, the opinion ultimately caused the clinician to find herself faced with a complaint to the state licensing board for practicing outside the competence of her profession.

SELECTING EXPERTS

The discussion on choosing witnesses in Chapter 4 focused on fact witnesses. Many of the same criteria apply for selecting expert witnesses: Is the witness credible? How good is his memory and recall? Will he be viewed as an objective information provider? This section highlights factors particular to selecting experts.

The level and type of expertise required depend on the type of expert evidence needed. For instance, making predictions about whether a sexual offender will commit another offense requires a higher level of experience than simply reporting on the general literature. Choosing an expert depends upon the nature of the legal and clinical issues, the expected roles of the expert, who is selecting the expert, and whether the witness would qualify as an expert according to the factors described above (specialized training, experience, etc.).

In some cases a clinician is asked to provide expert evidence simply because she has been working with a particular client. This testimony would be expert testimony based upon clinical knowledge rather than that drawn from a forensic evaluation. For example, Freida knows the Carveys very well from her family therapy with them. She can provide both fact and opinion evidence. She was working with Paula and Philip before litigation was contemplated, so they were not enticed to sway her assessments. However, Freida would need to testify about the limitations of her data, particularly focusing on how her data are drawn only from a clinical context. Her assessment may not have the breadth of information that might be obtained from a more comprehensive assessment.

In contrast, Evelyn was hired specifically to provide a custody evaluation, in light of impending litigation. In hiring Evelyn, Philip and Paula would be looking for a professional with a reputation for neutrality, fairness, objectivity, and independence, as well as a reputation as a competent, respected evaluator. Although hiring an evaluator may lead to a settlement, the parties hiring the evaluator should also be concerned about how the evaluator would provide evidence, should the case proceed to trial. Ideally, an expert witness should have no prior connection with the individuals involved in the dispute. The expert is hired for her expertise in forensic investigations and for ability to provide opinion evidence in a professional, credible manner.

The evidence of an expert hired by both parties tends to carry more weight than that of an expert hired by one party. A jointly hired expert avoids the possibility of dueling experts with conflicting opinions. Both parties are also more likely to cooperate with the expert, since both parties view the expert as an impartial professional.

If an interdisciplinary team has been working with a client, the attorney may decide to call only one or two members of the team as witnesses. Often, this decision is made according to which member of the team will have the greatest status (generally, the psychiatrist). However, the best person to provide the evidence may be the one who has had the most direct contact or has made the more critical observations. Even though Evelyn's supervisor may have better credentials, Evelyn is the one who conducted the home visits with the Carveys.

For some attorneys, the key characteristic sought in an expert is the ability to be a good educator. An effective expert is able to translate complex phenomena into language that can easily be understood. During preparation for a case, Lori may hire an expert to teach her about the current research examining how children are affected by exposure to child abuse. There may be research addressing the specific allegations raised in the present case. In such an instance, it would be appropriate for Lori to talk about the specific research and its applicability to the case before the court.

During the hearing, this expert may also be used to educate the tribunal on the same matters. An expert is helpful[8] to the court to the degree that she effectively communicates new and complex information into language that is easily understood by the judge and jury (if any). If an expert uses a lot of complicated jargon, the meaning of the information may be lost; alternatively, the judge may question whether the ex-

---

[8]We have used the concept of "helpful" in two different ways throughout this volume. In the context above, helpful means how experts can assist the court and reflects the everyday usage of the term. The other way "helpful" is used in this volume is to describe the legal concept of helpfulness (Shuman & Sales, 1998). In this context, helpful refers to the application of specific research finds to specific facts in a case. The greater the similarity between the factors in the research and the factors in the specific case, the greater the likelihood that the research results directly address the issues before the court.

pert really knows what she is talking about or whether she is trying to cover up weaknesses in her testimony. The expert needs to be able to explain herself in plain language, without losing technical accuracy or talking down to the tribunal. She must be well respected for her expertise, but not pretentious, biased, or dogmatic. She must be able to be authoritative and convincing, but also pleasant and easy to listen to (Cameron, 1995; Fradsham & Lamoureux, 1995).

When an attorney selects an expert, he will prefer someone he feels he can trust and with whom he can work This feeling may come from a prior working relationship or preliminary discussions with a new person. Different attorneys have different styles. An authoritarian attorney will prefer a clinician who provides her expertise as requested but does not try to assume a role in strategizing or directing the case. A collaborative attorney will want a clinician who will take a more active role in these matters. Sometimes, the clinician needs to develop trust before trying to participate as an equal partner.

While an attorney is assessing you as a potential expert, you should also be evaluating whether this is an attorney you want to work with: What is his reputation as a litigator? How does he treat clinicians? What position is he representing? How well can he communicate the intricacies of the law? Is he able to allay your fears about testifying? Is he willing and able to learn about your field of practice? Is he willing to incorporate your advice on matters within your expertise? If he decides to call you as a witness, will he allow you to answer truthfully, even if some of the information goes against his case? Given your style and how you see your role, consider whether the two of you are a good match. Think about whether the attorney has experience with cases involving your field of expertise. If not, you might suggest that the attorney work with a co-counsel with the required specialization to handle certain parts of the case (Tanay, 1978). Finally, are you competent to provide the services requested? If not, refer the attorney to someone who is more appropriate. Freida may be expert in the research addressing psychological causes of sexual aggression, but a physician may be needed to speak to physiological causes.

In cases where the tribunal assigns an expert, the tribunal usually relies upon the same professionals that it has used in other cases. The tribunal may have a certain roster of assessors or diagnosticians, or it may be affiliated with specific agencies (e.g., family court clinics, victim assistance programs, or psychiatric institutions). The most important criteria for the tribunal are generally the expert's level of expertise and the perceived impartiality of the expert. The expert must not have any monetary interest or investment in a particular outcome. For example, since Sam works for the child protection agency, the court could not ask him to provide an independent assessment in a child protection hearing.

To identify recognized experts in a particular field, attorneys investigate a number of sources: court-affiliated services, similar adjudications that have used experts, professional journals and books, public presentations, universities or other research centers, and professional associations (Barker & Branson, 1993). If you want attorneys to know of your expertise, you may need to speak for, write for, or join these types of organizations. To facilitate being hired as an expert, assemble a professional portfolio including your *curriculum vitae*, publications, sample reports, and transcripts of past evidence. If you have any biases or conflicts of interest, disclose these before you agree to work as an expert (e.g., if you have any past or present relationship with any of the parties to a litigation). An attorney may have contacted you because she suspected you would be sympathetic to her client's cause. Alternatively, she may be looking for someone who is untainted.

CONTRACT FOR SERVICES

A clinician may be retained as an expert by the tribunal, by one party, or by both parties to an action. If the tribunal retains the expert, then the contract for services is with the tribunal. More often, courts and other tribunals will order or recommend that the parties retain their own independent expert. Clinicians are sometimes engaged as witnesses without any explicit contract for services. To clarify your role and avoid any miscommunications, preferred practice is to use a written contract for services. A legally drafted retainer (service contract) will ensure that everyone's legal rights and responsibilities are covered. However, your own letter confirming the parameters of your services may be sufficient.

Initially, an attorney may contact you by telephone or letter to explore whether you are willing and able to provide services as an expert. You might suggest a face-to-face meeting to exchange information and to negotiate a contract for service. While an exchange of letters or telephone calls may be expedient, an in-person meeting will help both of you evaluate how effectively you can work together. Topics that should be discussed and outlined in the retainer or confirmation letter include the basic facts of the situation, the attorney's undertakings, your obligations, remuneration for your services, and contingencies (see Appendices A, B, C, and D).

In terms of the basic information, the attorney should spell out the name of the party engaging you, the names of other parties involved in the dispute, the presenting problems, the legal issues, the facts agreed upon, and the facts in dispute. In a refugee hearing, for example, you could be hired as a consultant for a refugee claimant, Sadru Nadji. The presenting problem is that Mr. Nadji's original application for refugee status has been turned down. The legal issue is how to interpret refugee legislation. The refugee board may agree that Mr. Nadji would not be in any physical danger if he were returned to his country of origin. The primary factual issue is whether the refugee has valid concerns regarding psychological torture.

While the attorney may be able to provide you with most of the factual information at the outset, consider what other information or assistance the attorney should undertake to provide for you on an ongoing basis. The refugee's attorney could undertake to provide the expert with documents filed with the refugee board, advise of any progress in settlement attempts or legal proceedings, and arrange for the refugee's voluntary participation in a psychological assessment. You could also ask the attorney for a more detailed analysis of the legal context of the case.

To clarify the parameters of your obligations, the contract or confirmation letter should provide details of the various services for which you are being retained (e.g., consultation, assessment, testifying, literature review, empirical research). If you are hired to conduct an assessment, the contract should specify the purpose of the investigation, procedures to be used for gathering information, the nature of the reports to be submitted, who will have access to the reports, and the time frames for information gathering and reporting (see Appendices A, B, C, and D). When the court appointed Evelyn, she forwarded her retainer agreement and informed consent information to each attorney with instructions to review the information with their clients, Paula and Philip. Her retainer stated that she was to provide an independent custody assessment examining areas pertaining to the psychological and social best interests of Debra. The methods and procedures used in her investigation would include use of parenting questionnaires, in-office interviews with the parties and the child, psychological test data, collateral interviews and record review, and direct behavioral observations of each parent with the minor child (Austin, 2000, 2001; Gould, 1998; Gould & Bell, 2000; Gould & Stahl, 2000). The scope of her evaluation would be guided by concerns relevant to issues before the court as stated in the court's order or indicated by a letter of agreement from the attorneys specifying the areas of concern to be addressed in the evaluation.[9] Evelyn would provide a custody evaluation by the end of 3 months, including recommendations for custody and access. Evelyn would give the report to the attorneys and the judge with the understanding that the report could be used in court and that Evelyn could be called to testify.

Some experts assist in investigation but are not called as witnesses. An expert hired by the aforementioned refugee might arrive at an unfavorable opinion. Although the attorney would not call this expert to testify at the refugee hearing, the information provided in the report could help the attorney know the case she is up against. The retainer agreement should not specify that the clinician is being hired to provide a particular opinion. This would not be ethical and would create an easy target for cross-examination. As an independent expert, you are not a client advocate. Unless you are court-appointed, the party(ies) who hired you can decide after you submit your findings whether to call you as a witness. If you believe an attorney is shopping around for a favorable expert, be careful about making any commitments that could damage your reputation in this case or in the future.

In some instances, such as closed mediation, both parties agree at the outset that the clinician's findings are not to be used in court or other adjudications. This encourages the parties to be frank and open in order to try to settle the conflict; the parties do not have to worry that the information could come back to haunt them if the case does not settle.

In addition to explaining your responsibilities, the retainer agreement could include what you will *not* do. Evelyn's retainer explained that she is not an expert in child abuse and that, if either parent had concerns about abuse, then the issues would be reported to child pro-

---

[9]See Amundson et al. (2000) and Gould (1999a, 1999b) for a fuller explanation of formulating questions that guide custody evaluations.

tection services to conduct an investigation. Evelyn would suspend her assessment until completion of the protection process.

Many cases involve more than one expert, either to provide corroborating evidence or to provide different types of expertise. If multiple experts are hired, your retainer agreement should define which expert is responsible for which information and functions. One expert may be designated as the coordinator of the work, who ensures that draft reports are shared before final reports are submitted. Each expert may be responsible to testify about the information he or she collected and interpreted. If you use a group model to conduct the evaluation, each party to the litigation needs to be clear about who is in charge. In the body of the report as well, as in oral testimony, the coordinator would need to clearly identify each group member's area of responsibility.

Sometimes an attorney will ask an expert to perform a preliminary assessment of the case and provide an oral report rather than a written report. In such cases, it is imperative that the expert and the attorney talk about the production of notes and other written material. The expert may be instructed not to take notes or produce any written materials so that there are no records that could be subject to a subpoena by the other party's attorney. Upon completion of the preliminary assessment, the expert may be asked to conduct a full evaluation or be told to stop work.

When you are hired by one side to perform an assessment, there may be times when you feel tension between the needs of a good evaluation and the needs of the attorney. There is no right and wrong way to approach this issue. You should be aware that the tension between the needs of the evaluator and the needs of the attorney can produce dynamic and challenging exchanges. For example, an attorney in a criminal case may ask you to interview some people while not interviewing other people. As an evaluation expert, you may feel strongly that you need to interview people from both groups. How you and the attorney negotiate these differences will often reflect upon the quality of your report. Imagine having to testify that the reason why you did not interview certain people was because the attorney who hired you said you couldn't interview them. How do you suppose the court would view your testimony? How do you suppose the court would view your independence and credibility?

No matter who hires you, you are in charge of how you conduct your evaluation. Make clear requests for information as well as access to collateral records and informants, and make those requests *in writing*. Although you are working for one side in a case, your ethical responsibility is to the court and the discovery of truth. Even if your evaluation never is presented to a court because the attorney views your results as harmful to his case, you should produce a document that reflects a properly conducted evaluation, not an evaluation that reflects what the attorney wanted.

Do not forget to negotiate terms of payment. If you are providing expert evidence pursuant to a subpoena, the amount that you can claim may be restricted to recovery of specific expenses and a nominal amount for your time.[10] If providing evidence is part of your agency role, such as in a parole department, you cannot claim remuneration in addition to your usual salary.

If you are hired as an independent expert, you will find that clinicians contracted as experts generally charge rates that are similar to or higher than their usual clinical rates. You should have a published list of charges. Some people charge one set of rates for in-office work and another set of rates for deposition and trial testimony. Your rates should reflect two factors: community standards and your level of expertise.[11]

Your retainer contract should also specify recoverable expenses (e.g., travel costs, overhead, secretarial support, research assistants, long-distance telephone charges, and postage). Note that it is common for clinicians who are operating in a forensic context to develop office business procedures that are based upon a legal model rather than a clinical model. Charges often include time for phone calls, note taking, consultation, and any other work-related operation that is associated with the legal case.

Terms of payment should depend on the time spent preparing for and participating in the legal process. Contingency arrangements (where payment depends on which party wins or whether the tribunal accepts the expert's testimony) may be unethical and can be used to destroy your credibility. An expert should be paid for her time, not for a particular outcome (see Appendix B).

Provide the attorney with an estimate of the time needed to con-

---

[10]In some cases, such as criminal trials, clinicians can be compelled to testify as fact witnesses without payment for services.

[11]See Ackerman and Ackerman (1997) for a discussion of hourly fees as well as total amount charged by child custody evaluators.

duct your assessment and to perform other services. During negotiations, the attorney should make you aware of any monetary constraints, particularly limitations on what the client can afford.[12] Since legal proceedings are costly even without fees for experts, consider a sliding-fee scale based upon ability to pay or pro bono (voluntary) services for appropriate clients.

A tough moral dilemma occurs when there are financial limits placed on the amount of time you put into a case. Do you accept a case for a fixed fee and perform all necessary functions, or do you accept a case and bill on an hourly basis, stopping work when the money runs out? Alternatively, do you negotiate a fee for a limited set of services? There are no clear answers about which pathway to take. It is never okay to provide a less competent work product because there is less money to be had. Each service you provide needs to be provided at the highest level of your professional ability. What you might need to do is limit how many services you provide, but never shortchange an attorney or party because they do not have the money to pay. Once you accept an assignment, you have an ethical responsibility to fulfill it to the highest level of your professional ability.

Adversarial proceedings can become intensely competitive and combative. They may leave clients feeling dissatisfied, in spite of the best efforts of the attorneys and clinicians involved. Recovering your fees at the end of the process may be problematic. As noted above, many clinicians who engage in forensic work adopt a legal paradigm for business practices. That paradigm entails an upfront retainer that enables you to bill your services in advance of your work. When the money runs out, you stop work until the retainer is replenished. Such business arrangements should be spelled out clearly in your retainer agreement.

Those clinicians who do not ask for their fees as a retainer up front normally opt to bill periodically. The contract should specify the time frame for payment and the interest penalty for late payments. Maintain time sheets for all contacts with clients or attorneys. Keep records for recoverable expenses. We believe it is always better to be paid in full prior to testifying. When you are paid in full, it renders moot the inevitable attempt to link the contents of your testimony to purportedly

---

[12]Occasionally, experts' fees are covered by the client's liability insurance or subsidized by legal aid. The scope of services covered by such plans is limited.

incentivized after-trial payments. "Doctor, isn't it true that full payment for your services will occur only after you complete your testimony? Isn't it also true that if you provide truthful testimony today, you might not collect all the fees due for your work here today?"

Ask the attorney about contingencies, such as the possibility of a settlement or delays. Your function may end at the time that initial conclusions are provided. If the case settles or there is insufficient basis to proceed, how will your services be terminated? If the attorney decides to use another expert in your place, can the other party call you to testify? If the case is delayed, will you be responsible for updating the assessment prior to the hearing?

The foregoing discussion deals with a broader spectrum of issues than most retainers actually encompass. Develop your own checklist or standard agreement to ensure that you deal with the issues that are most relevant to your situation. Ideally, have your personal attorney look over your retainer agreement.

DIRECT EXAMINATION

Most of the suggestions in Chapter 5 for oral testimony apply to not only fact witnesses but also expert witnesses. In this section we highlight four areas that apply specifically to expert witnesses: the elements of expert testimony; engaging the tribunal; providing opinions; and language with multiple meanings.

The Elements of Expert Testimony

Direct examination should be presented in a logical, step-by-step fashion. As noted earlier, the first stage of the examination is qualifying the witness as an expert. The attorney will take you through your *curriculum vitae*, generally in chronological order, and highlight the information that is most relevant to the types of opinions you will provide. Upon being qualified, your attorney will ask you to describe when and how you became involved in the case. To lay the basis for your findings and recommendations, describe your information-gathering process (e.g., where, when, and how you interviewed each person). If you used any diagnostic or assessment tools, explain their purpose, how they were administered, and the reliability of these tools. Clarify whether you followed your discipline's generally accepted standards for gathering information. If you did not follow these standards, then explain why (the case at hand may not have been a standard case, or you may have had to deal with a particularly resistant client).

Once you have identified the sources of your information, present your factual findings. These findings could include the perspectives and wishes of the people interviewed, interpretation of data from your psychological and psychosocial testing, interviews with collateral information sources that may include other clinicians, and direct observations of the subjects of the case (in a custody case, this would be each parent with the child). Your factual findings form the foundation for the next element of your testimony, your expert opinions. Opinion evidence includes explanations of psychological and psychosocial phenomena, interpretations of the data collected, predictions based upon research findings, and predictions based upon your judgment as an experienced clinician.

Each opinion needs to be connected with a theoretical and factual foundation. Move from general to specific; outline what the general theory is, how the current independent data sources support or do not support different perspectives, and how you have chosen to interpret the data to support an opinion that favors a particular recommendation. You may then be asked to discuss each of your recommendations and conclusions in light of the described data.

To preempt criticisms that could be raised in cross-examination, it is usually a good idea to identify possible gaps or inconsistencies in your facts and opinions. You may be able to explain how you dealt with these problems. In some cases, you may have to admit that your information gathering, theory, or research has certain weaknesses. After all, behavioral and social science disciplines are inexact sciences (Chisholm & McNaughton, 1990; Watson, 1978).

Your written report (discussed in Chapter 8) could be entered as an exhibit. During the oral examination, you would summarize your report and highlight important information. Remember, during the direct examination, you will most likely be asked open-ended questions. Be prepared to go through your information in detail without too many prompts from the attorney. There are some attorneys who like to conduct a direct examination with specific closed-ended questions. Preparation is the key to successful testimony in such cases.

Engaging the Tribunal

As an expert witness, *how* you present is just as important as *what* you present. Building a positive rapport with the tribunal should begin with your first impression and continue throughout your testimony. A frequent mistake is that clinicians begin their testimony with an *unduly dry* recitation of their educational and professional achievements.

To be interesting, you should convey your story in an interesting manner. Think about the best teacher that you have ever had and what made that person a good teacher. Effective educators use many different methods of presentation. Narrative is an important element in effective education. Sometimes, the use of graphics or visual devices may enhance understanding and make the information more memorable.

Some jurisdictions permit greater creativity than others. For example, some jurisdictions may allow Freida to use videotapes, live sculpting,[13] or psychodrama to illustrate family relationships. In other jurisdictions the witness may be limited to verbal reports—within which may be used imagery, metaphors, and analogies to help bring the information to life! In presenting his child protection assessment, Sam conveyed a vivid picture of Debra rather than a sterile report on an anonymous child in need of protection. He drew specific connections between child welfare theory and Debra's personal needs. She was not in court, so he brought along photographs.

Vary the format of your answers and use pronouns purposefully. Stating, "From psychological research on sexual abuse, *we* understand that . . . " tends to emphasize that this information is generally understood. In contrast, stating, "From my review of research on sexual abuse, *I* understand that . . . " tends to personalize the testimony. Some subtleties, perhaps not so noticeable during oral testimony, may carry more weight in the proceeding's transcript (Brodsky, 1991).

A common mistake among experts is that they come across as patronizing or disrespectful. For the most part, experts have good intentions, but they may be unaware of how their behavior is interpreted.

---

[13]Live sculpting and psychodrama refer to methods of demonstrating interactions between people. Participants act out a situation so that observers and participants can gain a more personal understanding of the dynamics.

Avoid flippant and defensive reactions. Expressing frustration with a questioner who does not seem to understand your answers may come across as arrogant. Correcting a questioner who mispronounces technical terms may sound condescending. Criticism of other experts could be interpreted as disdain. To function as an effective educator, demonstrate patience with those who are learning. Be careful not to embarrass learners about areas beyond their current knowledge. All of us have something to learn. When we feel safe and respected, we are more open to learning.

Providing Opinions

Qualifying as an expert witness allows you to put your opinions on the record. However, you are probably interested not only in being heard but also in influencing the decisions to be made. Opinions based on intuition or gut reaction generally carry little weight. To maximize the influence of your opinions, present them with confidence and base them on factual evidence and persuasive theory.

Do not disguise a personal or political belief as scientific knowledge (Wasyliw, Cavanaugh, & Rogers, 1985). Consider the impact of corporal punishment on child development. Many clinicians have a strong negative view, based on moral beliefs and personal values, on the appropriateness of corporal punishment. To be an effective expert witness, be prepared to discuss the research about use of corporal punishment, its limitations, and potential usefulness. In adjudicative processes, personal beliefs are weak substitutes for empirical evidence.

While some clinicians come across as arrogant, others err by using wishy-washy language and self-deprecating remarks. "I'm just a psychologist, but if you really want my opinion, I think that Philip may not have been very nice to Debra. But then again, maybe. . . . " What is the likelihood that Debra was abused, and what information supports that conclusion? Present your information with confidence. Couch your opinions in terms of their probability, as supported by the knowledge in your field. "Seventy-five percent of children with Debra's pattern of sleep disturbances reported having experienced sexual abuse." Clinical assessments often require some level of subjective opinion. You do not need 100% certainty, or any other specific percentage, to express an opinion. "Based on the facts outlined in my report, within a reasonable degree of psychological certainty,[14] I concluded that Debra was sexually abused." If confident in a belief, don't waiver. If not, admit the information is tentative. A qualified opinion is better than a misleading opinion or no opinion at all.

Provide your opinions with confidence. Still, you should distinguish between confidence and certainty. You may feel very confident about the opinion you offer the court while at the same time providing information to the Court that you are uncertain about the scientific foundation for the conclusions.

When offering expert opinion about *scientific information*, you need to provide the court with an understanding of the research that supports your conclusions. On the other hand, if you are offering expert opinion about a *clinical issue*, the standard of admissible evidence may be somewhat lower (Shuman & Sales, 1998). For example, claims based on research or theory should be backed up by current literature and research. In the example above, you may need to be prepared with appropriate research to answer the question "How do you know corporal punishment is harmful?" Bring an annotated bibliography of current and accepted literature that provides research on both sides of the issue. Be prepared to explain competing ideas in the literature and how your interpretation in this particular case is more compelling than any other interpretation. Be prepared to summarize the methods and findings of these studies as well as their limitations. When offering an opinion on a clinical issue (such as your assessment of Debra's ability to cope with her parent's divorce), your opinion should be supported by your clinical experience and judgment, though research evidence is also a useful plus.

The basis of your opinion may be more important than the opinion itself since the tribunal needs a basis upon which to evaluate, accept, or reject your evidence. Use concrete, specific, and observable facts. Stay away from such statements as "Paula is neglectful." There are two problems with testimony such as this. The first is that concluding that Paula is neglectful might be tantamount to addressing the ultimate issue to be decided in the case, which is the job of the judge (or jury), not the witness. The second is that the term "neglectful" is an interpretative state-

---

[14]For an expert who is not a psychologist, this phrase should be adapted to fit the person's discipline: for example, "sociological certainty" or "criminological certainty."

ment that does not provide a clear description of behaviors that are of concern. It would be better if Evelyn could simply provide facts that support this conclusion. "When I arrived at the house, Debra was alone in the basement, playing with the power saw and drill, while I observed Paula to be watching television, occasionally hollering down to Debra to 'be a good girl.' " These facts beg the tribunal to draw its own conclusions. By focusing on the factual basis rather than the actual opinion, you also avoid problems with the ultimate issue doctrine, described earlier. Inexperienced clinician-witnesses are particularly prone to stating conclusions without factual support. If you cannot identify observable facts to support your opinion, then consider whether it is well founded. You might be setting yourself up for a difficult cross-examination.

Opinions can be based on direct observations, case records, testimony presented in the hearing, hypothetical situations,[15] your own research, or professional literature. If you base your opinion on facts from your observations or readings of the case file, it is generally better to lay the factual foundation for your opinions first. "Based upon the hospital records supplied to me, Mr. Carvey admits that he has not gone a day without drinking alcohol during the past 6 years. When he wakes up in the morning, he feels nauseous and his hands shake. These behaviors are similar to those reported in the literature as characteristic of people who are physically addicted to alcohol. Therefore, based upon this review of records and current behavioral science literature, it is my opinion that Mr. Carvey is physically addicted to alcohol." The witness might go on to explain the nature of physical addiction and how it is defined by withdrawal effects. If you base an opinion on facts that are in the records, make sure that you have all of the facts. Nausea and shakiness can be caused by a variety of conditions. For example, did you happen to know that Mr. Carvey has multiple sclerosis?

If you lack direct knowledge about a clinical situation, you might be asked for an opinion based on a hypothetical situation. "Assuming that these facts are true, do you have an opinion? What is your opinion? What is the basis for your opinion?" In preparing for the case, review the hypothetical facts with the attorney who will present them. The hy-

---

[15]For example, Lori asks a child psychologist who has not seen any of the Carveys and has not heard any of the trial proceedings to provide an opinion about a hypothetical situation that closely resembles the picture of the Carveys that Lori has led in evidence.

pothetical facts could be written down to ensure that they are accurately repeated during the direct examination.

Another method for introducing expert opinions is to call witnesses with factual information and have the expert listen to their testimony before calling the expert to testify. This approach can be tricky since the facts presented are not necessarily the facts proven. The expert witness may still have to respond to a hypothetical question. "Assuming Sam's testimony was true, do you have an opinion within a reasonable degree of psychological certainty?"

Using multiple sources of information corroborates your evidence, giving it greater credibility (Austin, 2001). Corroboration is akin to the concept of triangulation in qualitative research (LeCompte & Schensul, 1999). Evelyn ratified the information gathered from personal interviews by reviewing prior assessments, by observing Debra's interaction with her parents, and by talking with people who have had direct observational knowledge of Debra's parenting such as teachers, coaches, and youth counselors. Our expert on refugees conducted a literature review on the causes and effects of psychological torture. He found that prior research was consistent with his own findings.

To enhance the credibility of your opinion, describe the thought processes that led you to your opinion. Identifying the pros and cons of your opinion will demonstrate that you have considered alternative possibilities before arriving at your conclusion. When you analyze your opinion, consider other possible hypotheses, options, and variables. A balanced assessment is more believable than one deliberately limited to favorable data.

Language with Multiple Meanings

Communications in legal proceedings can be complicated by the fact that people come from different cultures: the dominant culture in the community, legal culture, professional clinical culture, and the cultures of minority participants in the process, to name a few. Each profession and each culture has its own language, even if everyone seems to be speaking English. In your role of expert-as-educator, you need to be able to adapt your language to communicate effectively with various participants (e.g., the decision makers, the attorneys, the parties, and the broader public).

During your preparation, find out who your target audience is. If the decision makers have a background in your field, use of technical language may be appropriate. If you come from a different culture than some of the participants, how familiar are you with their culture and patterns of communication? If you are not very familiar, consider using a cultural interpreter to help you prepare for your testimony.

Legal definitions of particular words can vary significantly from what a clinician or layperson might expect. If a piece of legislation states that a cat is a dog, then, for the purposes outlined in the legislation, a cat is a dog. Drug legislation provides an interesting illustration of this type of legal fiction. The legislation establishes criminal offenses for possessing or trafficking in narcotics. Narcotics are then listed. Substance abuse clinicians will note that a narcotic is a sleep-inducing substance. According to the legal definition, however, narcotics include a number of stimulants. The legal definition also excludes certain drugs that, in pharmacological terms, are narcotics. If you are asked whether your client used narcotics, how do you respond?

Clinicians too have their own peculiar definitions. The *Diagnostic and Statistical Manual of Mental Disorders* (American Psychiatric Association, 2000) provides psychiatrists with specific criteria to diagnose mental disorders. In earlier editions the manual offered a definition for the term "psychopath." In more recent editions "psychopath" was deleted and the term "sociopath" was added. Does this mean we have no more psychopaths? Other conditions have remained the same but have different definitions. Perhaps this is not so peculiar, since all languages evolve. Reciting a DSM definition in order to educate the court about a mental disorder may not provide sufficient information for the court decision makers to really understand the disorder. Explaining the term in concrete and specific language may be more helpful than relying on the technical definitions.

Problems tend to arise when people are not sure about the language others are using. If an attorney asked you about a client's mental capacity, would you know that he is referring to a term that has a specific legal meaning? In fact, it may have several meanings. Is the attorney asking whether the client has the capacity to enter into a will, whether the client has the capacity to choose or deny medical treatment, or whether the person is legally competent to stand trial? The requirements for mental capacity differ depending on the legal issues at stake. As you are exposed to particular areas of law, you will become more familiar with legal concepts that relate to your field of practice. It is critical to discuss language issues with your attorney during the preparation stage. In some situations, the attorney may suggest that you avoid use of language with legal definitions. In other situations, she may encourage you to use legal terminology. If you do, make sure that you are well informed about its meaning.[16]

During the hearing, listen carefully for what is being asked. "What makes you believe that Debra is in need of protection?" The phrase "in need of protection" may have a specific legal meaning. When you respond to this type of question, break down the legal constructs into plain language components and translate the legal question into observables. "In need of protection" refers to sexual, physical, or emotional abuse and neglect. If you are basing your opinion that Debra needs protection because you believe there was sexual abuse, you need to state what you observed that constituted sexual abuse.

You may also need to understand the relationship between the diagnostic categories and standards used for different legal issues. In criminal law, an accused person may claim that he is not guilty by reason of mental disorder (popularly known as an insanity defense). An expert witness who specializes in such cases must be familiar not only with the psychiatric criteria for diagnosing a mental disorder but also with the specific legal criteria for relieving an accused person of criminal responsibility. Given the challenges of using different sets of terminology, it is almost as if the expert needs to be multilingual.

CROSS-EXAMINATION

As with fact witnesses, thorough preparation and a sound direct examination are the best defense for an expert witness during cross-examination. Expert witnesses are typically the most challenging witnesses to cross-examine. They have expertise that goes beyond that of the cross-examining attorney, giving the expert an informational advantage. An opposing attorney may choose not to cross-examine, particularly if the expert has shown that she is clinically and forensically competent and skilled at providing testimony. Expect that at least part of your testi-

---

[16]Consistent use of terminology is vital. Use the same words to describe the same concepts and use different words to describe different concepts. If you switch from talking about "abuse" to "assault" or "mistreatment," note that each term has different connotations.

mony will be weakened in cross-examination and realize that perfect expert testimony is an unrealistic goal.

The primary focuses for cross-examination of an expert may be to challenge the expert's qualifications or impartiality, as well as the factual and theoretical basis of his opinions.

Challenging Qualifications

If an opposing attorney challenges your qualifications, such a challenge is generally made when you initially present your qualifications rather than after you have testified. That way, if you do not qualify as an expert, there is no need to go through your testimony. Even if you are admitted as a qualified expert, opposing attorneys can use cross-examination to try to narrow the scope of your expertise or to challenge your overall credibility. For instance, an attorney might challenge a social worker in a supervisory role for not having any recent direct practice with clients (Brodsky, 1991). Remember, the key to responding to cross-examination is to maintain your composure and respond in a nondefensive manner. Demonstrate your knowledge of relevant literature and practice issues. Confirm your expertise with confidence. Admit your limitations.

Be careful about questions that go beyond your expertise or statutory authority. In some jurisdictions, for example, only certain regulated professionals are allowed to provide a clinical diagnosis. If you are asked a question beyond your expertise or authority, do not be embarrassed to say that you are not qualified or authorized to provide such an opinion. This approach is much safer than allowing the attorney to lead you "down a garden path."

Challenging Impartiality

The opposing attorney may challenge your impartiality by suggesting bias in your information gathering, assessment process, report, or oral testimony. Even if you feel attacked, cooperate with the attorney, as cooperation will enhance your appearance of honesty and neutrality.

Some attorneys try to imply bias by asking the expert who is paying him. As recommended in Chapter 5, be frank about whether you have been paid for your consultation or your court appearance. Note that *you are being paid for your time, not for stating a particular opinion.* If you make your living as an expert witness, you may be questioned about this. If you always appear on behalf of a particular type of disputant (e.g., accused hate mongers), you risk being painted as biased in favor of that party. When Sam is called as an expert witness, he always represents the child protection agency. Although he always represents the same party, he can note that he does not always come to the same conclusion.

Expert witnesses, like all people, have biases. We are personally biased against hate mongering. Does that mean we cannot be objective in a case where someone is accused of this? If you are asked whether you have a bias about what should happen in a case, state your beliefs, based on your observations and expertise. The important issue is not whether you have a bias after your assessment but whether you brought preexisting biases with you and whether they affected your approach to the task.

Accusations of racial or cultural bias are difficult to handle. Asserting that you are not prejudiced can come across as defensive. Consider whether you may have had such prejudices and what (if anything) you did to deal with them. Many assessment tools used by clinicians do have inherent biases. Mainstreaming children from ethnic minorities into special education, for example, has been challenged on the basis of cultural bias. Is there any literature that indicates whether the assessment procedures incur cultural biases or that supports ways to avoid such biases?

Challenging Factual Bases

If you were responsible for gathering information to inform your assessment, cross-examination could be used to challenge the thoroughness of your investigation—whether or not you followed reasonable standards from your discipline—and the strength of the information you relied upon. Be familiar with standards for gathering information, including the recent literature, published protocols established by your agencies or associations, and current training and textbooks. If you have not followed established standards, be prepared to deal with questions about how you deviated and why? Be prepared to discuss how your approach provides a more thorough or more competent evaluation than if you followed established or conventional protocols.

If an expert is called to provide factual information and the client himself is not called to testify on his own behalf, the tribunal may wonder why the client is not taking the stand. A client may not be called to testify in order to protect the individual from difficult or embarrassing situations. Alternatively, the individual may not be a "good witness" due to uneasiness in public situations, limited communication skills, or poor memory. Some criminal courts have special rules permitting hearsay evidence to be heard from a clinician when a child or other victim has an impediment to testifying. Be aware that cross-examination may be used to suggest that your side is trying to hide something by not calling this witness. If there is a good reason that the person is not being called, it may be useful to disclose this reason. Before you disclose such information, be certain that the attorney wants you to provide such information to the court. Of course, even if the attorney does not want you to disclose such information, once you take the stand, you may be compelled to answer that question unless the attorney successfully objects to it.

In situations where you are asked to base your opinions on hypothetical situations or the reports of others, you have less control over the factual basis of your evidence. If you based your original opinion on a hypothetical set of facts, the attorney may ask if your opinion would be different if there were additional facts (Cameron, 1995). The additional facts may seem incredulous and you may have trouble accepting them. Remember that these facts are hypothetical. When you assume them, you are not agreeing with them. "The situation you are asking me to assume seems unlikely and is very different from that to which I have just offered testimony. However, if you would like me to include these variables in a different hypothetical situation, my opinion about this different circumstance would be . . . " In order for your opinion to be used in the final adjudication, of course, the assumptions in the opposing attorney's version of the hypothetical would need to be proven.

If you received your facts from a secondhand source, you could be asked, "You weren't there when the riot erupted, so how do you know what happened?" Good question. A possible answer is: "That is correct. I was not there. I based my assessment on the reports of my associate, Dr. Johanna Perez." The rules of hearsay are relaxed somewhat for experts who have gathered information for an assessment. The court may look at whether the expert used standard methods and sources of information rather than require that court standards of admissibility be met. For example, is it common practice for a psychiatrist to rely on psychometric tests administered by a psychologist? If the factual basis of the assessment is in issue, the tribunal may require that the people who informed the expert take the stand personally so that they can be subject to live examination and cross-examination. The tribunal might also consider whether the source was likely to be honest. During an assessment, Paula might have an incentive to mislead Evelyn, so Paula's statements to Evelyn would be suspect. In contrast, an independent source such as Freida has no stake in the outcome and no personal reason to mislead Evelyn. Freida's statements might be trusted.

There is no need to prove every single fact that the expert said she relied upon. The weight given to an opinion, however, will depend on how well the factual basis underlying the opinion can be proven. To ensure that your opinions are given due weight, find out what the facts are before the hearing and whether evidence can be presented to prove those facts. You do not want to have your opinions undermined during cross-examination because the factual basis cannot be proven.

Challenging Theoretical Bases

Technically, if an expert quotes someone else's research or articles, that information is hearsay evidence. Tribunals will generally allow an expert to quote other people's work, provided that the work is well documented. The witness should be able to produce copies of the work, even though they may not be requested. If you are relying on literature for the theoretical basis of your opinion, use the original sources of information (i.e., the original theorist or the report of the original researchers). Your sources could easily be challenged if you rely on secondhand sources such as literature reviews or abstracts. How do you know the review or the abstract is accurate?

Theory can be challenged on the grounds that it is dated, unreliable, or invalid. To defend against these claims, be thoroughly familiar with the research you are relying upon, as well as research that may go against your case. You may be asked, "Is the theory you used the only theory in current use?" Explain that there are other theories and why you chose to rely on this particular one. The weight attributed to your opinions will depend on a number of factors: Does the literature support your opinion? Are your opinions consistent with scientific principles? Are your inferences logical? Are the assumptions reasonable? Is your process of reasoning consistent, explainable, objective, and defensible (Myers, 1993)?

If you rely on part of a book or article, you may be cross-examined on the whole work. If a book is entered as an exhibit, you generally need to adopt the opinion of the book. If you agree with parts of the book and disagree with other parts of the book, be prepared to discuss the reasons why you disagree with aspects of the work. Having research to back up your position is always helpful. You may be cross-examined on any book that you refer to or that you admit is authoritative. As part of your preparation, ask your attorney which other experts will be called, what issues may arise, and what other literature they will likely introduce. Ensure that you are familiar with this literature and how it relates to your evidence.

If you are confronted with obscure references or quotations provided out of context, feel free to ask to see the book or reference. You might also want to ask the attorney to read the relevant quote so that you can respond to it. Be honest if you have not read a particular book or article (Watson, 1978). You cannot be questioned about readings or authors with which you are unfamiliar.

Another method of challenging expert evidence is to identify inconsistent statements. These inconsistencies could arise within your own testimony, between what you said on the stand and what you said previously, or between your testimony and information from others (including other witnesses, theorists, researchers, or common belief). If Sam has a theory about neglect that is inconsistent with common belief, he will have an uphill battle to prove his theory. Some people still believe that the Earth is flat. If Sam's assessment practices went against what is said in traditional literature, he would need strong proof to demonstrate that his practices are valid or he would have to provide a more persuasive work product for the court.

The cross-examining attorney may try to get mileage from the fact that you are not perfect, even if the inconsistency is not crucial to your overall testimony. Do not get flustered. Consider the possibility that you may be wrong (e.g., you may have made an error in judgment or missed a piece of information that the other side has uncovered and brought to your attention). Admit a mistake rather than try to cover it up. If you have changed your opinion from a prior time, explain why you changed it. Try to convey professionalism and confidence with your current statements. Your research may be more recent or more rigorous than the other research quoted. Explain the methodological soundness of your research in terms that the tribunal can comprehend.

If the apparent inconsistency is not real, you may be able to clarify your statements or distinguish the contexts. "In the first case, I was quoted as supporting Theory X. In this case, I am relying on Theory Y. That is because the first case involved heroin abuse, and in this case Philip has been abusing cocaine." Your testimony is more credible if you correct past inconsistencies rather than avoid them or deal with them grudgingly. You might try to explain the inconsistencies during the direct examination to avoid the appearance that you are trying to hide something. If cross-examination has damaged your testimony, some of this damage may be reparable in the redirect. For example, your attorney can ask you to explain apparent inconsistencies or fill in some of the missing context.

Given that anything you say (or write) can be used against you in a future legal proceeding, be careful about how you express yourself publicly. Expressing controversial views may come back to haunt you.

Proof in law is different from scientific proof, although scientific methods and statistical probabilities are helpful in establishing proof in law. In law, the tribunal ultimately assesses whether the appropriate legal standard has been met. Consider an expert who is asked, "Are you certain, beyond a reasonable doubt?" The expert should use her own terms to describe her level of certainty about a particular opinion rather than the terminology that describes the legal standard of proof required. The language of a clinician professional might be "within a reasonable degree of certainty." This avoids using the legal term "reasonable doubt." You want to convey confidence; however, you do not want to overstate your certainty since this could hurt your credibility. It all goes back to just being honest.

RELIABILITY AND VALIDITY

One of the greatest challenges for both individual clinicians and the clinical professions is to demonstrate the reliability and validity of clinical theory and research. In the terminology of qualitative research, how do we know that certain information is trustworthy? In legal terminology, how do we know that the information is credible? In some fields that clinicians draw from, there is a considerable foundation of research (e.g., learning theory or attachment theory). In other fields, there is only theoretical support or a weak foundation of empirical research. There is a long-standing debate, for instance, about the accuracy of information recalled by a witness under hypnosis (Swenson, 1997).[17] The human sciences are riddled with uncertainties and unfathomable possibilities.

Although an expert witness should have a thorough understanding of the various types of validity and reliability, the depth of information required in this area goes beyond the scope of this volume (Kassin, Tubb, Hosch, & Memon, 2001). If you need to enhance your research knowledge, numerous good texts and courses offered through universities and research institutes are available.

You need to know research methods well enough to be able to translate them into terms that can be understood by people who have not read the text or taken university research courses. For example, if you were giving evidence about the validity of a personality test, you could explain validity as, briefly: "Does the test measure what it is intended to measure?" Similarly, for a simple explanation of reliability: "Would another clinician using the same test come up with a similar finding?" Provide concrete examples to illustrate these concepts. As noted earlier, demonstrations are also useful educational devices. If you want to demonstrate the statistical principles of probability and the independence of events, you could use the simple toss of a coin. "What is the probability of getting heads? (Flip a coin.) It came up heads. What is the probability that it will come up heads the next time?"

During cross-examination of your testimony, the validity and reliability of your expert testimony could be challenged in terms of the following aspects:

- Assumptions underlying the theory or research methods
- Methodological criticism
- Inconsistencies between different research or articles
- Researcher bias
- Level of uncertainty[18]

---

[17]Similarly, the accuracy of polygraphs (lie detectors) has spawned much psychological research and debate. You may wish to consult the entire December 1998 issue of *Psychology, Public Policy and Law* for a discussion of legal and psychological issues relating to memory.

[18]See the entire March 1999 issue of *Psychology, Public Policy and Law*, which addresses the admissibility of behavioral and social science evidence.

Consider a commission of inquiry into the existence of racial discrimination in a school system. How would we know that discrimination exists? Is there sufficient research to answer this type of question? Experts are sometimes asked for information to help resolve public policy issues, but in certain areas of inquiry the available research knowledge is unreliable or uncertain. Clinicians should not get caught up in a political dispute and try to convey expert knowledge in an area when none exists. This does not mean that experts should not testify when conflicting research findings or legitimate differences of professional opinion exist. Clinicians should present the knowledge that exists, including areas of uncertainty or controversy.

Although clinicians are frequently called as experts to provide assessments, much debate surrounds what expert evidence should be admitted, how it should be used, and whether it is reliable and valid (Shuman & Sales, 1998). Tests, measures, procedures, and concepts from psychology, social work, and related disciplines may be subjected to challenges before a court accepts testimony based upon these tests, measures, procedures, or concepts. Such challenges often change over time. The two most common challenges—the *Frye* challenge and the *Daubert* challenge—are based upon important legal decisions. The *Frye* (1993) test suggests that expert evidence is only admissible if it is based upon a theory or research finding that has "general acceptance in the particular field in which it belongs." The *Daubert* (1993) challenge suggests that expert evidence must be based on information that is not only reliable and valid but also obtained through sound scientific methods. A third type of challenge is called a relevancy analysis. A fourth type of challenge is called a helpfulness challenge.

Each type of challenge has the same primary goal. The challenge examines whether the proffered method, procedure, or concept will provide reliable, relevant, and helpful information that can be useful to the trier of fact.

Some of these tools, such as the MMPI-2, Wechsler scales, the Rorschach, and the MCMI-III, have been subject to the court's scrutiny, and each has been determined to be a scientific instrument within the legal meaning of that term (McCann & Dyer, 1996; Pope, Butcher, & Seelen, 2000). Other tools have been determined to have too inadequate a scientific foundation to be admissible as a scientific instrument, for example, the House–Tree–Person or Sentence Completion Test (Lilienfeld, Wood, & Grab, 2000).

When conducting an assessment for legal purposes, consider using methods and definitions that have been accepted in precedent cases. For example, in several jurisdictions, the concept of Parental Alienation Syndrome is inadmissible, yet one can present testimony about alienation dynamics. The issue with this concept is that, because the legal definition of a syndrome is often judged not to have been met, testimony about Parental Alienation Syndrome is deemed inadmissible. Testimony about behaviors that appear to characterize alienation dynamics may be admissible. Legal definitions drawn from case law precedents may exist about several important psychological and social phenomena. There are legal definitions for "battered wife syndrome" that provide a listing of symptoms that have been legally recognized as constituting this condition. There are federal as well as state definitions for the "best interests of the child." There are psychological and social dimensions drawn from case law when examining a parent's request to relocate away from the noncustodial parent.

While tribunals are generally willing to rely on diagnostic tools for assessment purposes, tribunals generally have much less confidence in their use for predictive purposes. A tribunal is likely to have little difficulty accepting evidence, for example, based on a diagnostic tool used to assess whether Philip suffered from a mental illness. On the other hand, a tribunal will tend to be more skeptical about use of a diagnostic tool that purports to predict Philip's risk of reoffending. The question raised by the court should be whether there is any proof to show that experts are any better at predicting behavior than anyone else. If the answer is yes, then you must show how the research provides a reliable, relevant, and helpful set of predictions to be used by the court in its decision making.

To demonstrate that they can predict better than lay witnesses, clinicians need to show that their opinions reflect more than just personal values or speculative beliefs. It is easy for biases to creep into an assessment. During a custody evaluation, Evelyn might find that Philip is more cooperative than Paula and that Philip is more amenable to family therapy. Evelyn could easily interpret this finding in a way that supports Philip's claim for custody. But how does Evelyn know that these factors will make Philip a better custodial parent? Is she biased by her attitude toward Paula's resistance?[19] Maybe Paula does not need psychotherapy. Is Philip putting on a show for Evelyn, trying to look good so as to obtain a favorable assessment? Evelyn needs to be aware of her potential biases. Research literature might suggest questions that help to identify the possibility of faking (or dissimilation) by a client. An assessment instrument that Evelyn is using may have ways to identify risks of deception.

Expert witnesses are not expected to be able to predict with 100% certainty. Expert opinions based upon useful research may provide helpful information to a court even if the opinion is framed as a statement of probability rather than an absolute certainty (Chisholm & McNaughton, 1990).

---

[19]When you interview a client for an assessment, the assessment may cause a client to be guarded. This reaction is natural. It is the situation that is not normal (Chisholm & McNaughton, 1990). Note whether the client's reaction is enduring or reactive. Is the client's responsiveness affected by the climate you have established during your interview?

Chapter 8

Documentary Evidence

Although much of our discussion has focused on clinicians called to produce oral evidence, in recent years many types of legal proceedings have tended to rely more and more heavily on written evidence. For tribunals, the primary advantage of adjudicating on the basis of documentary evidence is speed, oral testimony being far more time-consuming than compiling written evidence. Written evidence also tends to be more focused than *viva voce* (live voice). Additionally, documentary processes do not depend on the ability to get all of the parties and decision makers in the same room at the same time. Some clinicians prefer written evidence because they do not have to perform at a public hearing and are not subjected to on-the-spot cross-examination. Clinicians may also feel more comfortable with the narrative character of documentary evidence, in contrast with the question-and-answer format of oral evidence. Among the drawbacks for clinicians are the time it takes to prepare documents and the inability to gauge how the decision makers are taking in the information. On the stand, at least a witness can perceive what types of evidence and manner of presentation seem most interesting to the decision maker(s).

In most legal proceedings a combination of written and oral evidence is used. For example, when Lori initiated divorce proceedings, she had to file a petition, or legal application for the divorce, outlining the grounds for the application. Lori might file written evidence from Freida with the application. Freida has a lot invested in what goes down on paper, because she is committed to certain facts and positions even though it is early in the legal process. It would hard for her to retract any statements made, particularly during any oral cross-examination, because inconsistent statements could discredit her decisiveness, honesty, or competence. On the other hand, effective written evidence can be used to corroborate and strengthen her oral testimony.

In some situations clinicians feel that the need to make a strong case for their position means they should not include disconfirming information in the written evidence. A parole officer who is recommending that parole be withdrawn might be inclined to include only negative information about the parolee. On the stand, the same officer might feel freer to provide balanced testimony about the parolee. In most instances, balanced information is preferable, regardless of whether the evidence is oral or written. Balance demonstrates that the witness is objective. Further, inclusion of positive information is likely to leave the client feeling better about the process and the clinician. Clinicians who hope or need to continue to work with a client following adjudication do not want to win the case and lose the person.

In this chapter, we deal with three types of documentary evidence: affidavits, reports, and exhibits. The following section describes each of these types of evidence. We then outline the key elements of reports and provide suggestions for reviewing them. The final section revisits the issue of language and how to be careful about what you put in writing.

TYPES OF DOCUMENTARY EVIDENCE

Affidavits

Affidavits are written statements that are sworn to or affirmed by a deponent, the person who has knowledge of the information contained in the affidavit (See Appendix E for a sample). Certain legal processes require that affidavits be witnessed by an attorney or a notary public. If a party wants to enter an affidavit into the records for a hearing, the affidavit must satisfy the rules of admissibility for that tribunal. For example, because of the rules against hearsay, the information should come primarily from the deponent's direct knowledge and beliefs. If an affidavit contains second-hand information, the source of the information should be stated: "I am advised by psychologist Fern Richards, PsyD, and do verily believe . . . " If the other party to the proceeding does not contest this information, then the tribunal may rely upon it. If the other party does contest it, then proof of Dr. Richards's information would have to come from her own testimony or affidavit. Tribunals normally recognize that mental health professionals often work as a team and that they should allow one professional to present all of the team's information in one document. Rather than paraphrase a coprofessional's report, another option is to attach the other professional's report as an exhibit to the affidavit.

Affidavits often require very specific information and formatting. For example, since an affidavit consists of personal observations, it should be written in the first-person singular voice (i.e., using "I" statements rather than "we," "the agency," or "the worker"). Each statement in an affidavit is written as a separately numbered paragraph, for ease of reference at a hearing.[1] Attorneys frequently take responsibility for drafting affidavits. However, a clinician who has been involved in a number of similar cases may be able to draft her own, subject to review by an attorney or supervisor. Do not hesitate to ask attorneys or court clerks for sample affidavits, if needed, and other assistance. Even if an attorney drafts your affidavit, prepare a detailed written summary of your information to use as the basis for the affidavit. Before swearing to or affirming an affidavit, read it carefully. Do not be embarrassed or hesitant to suggest changes for greater clarity and accuracy. You may have additional information, or you may have questions about the wording and its legal significance.

If you are preparing an affidavit that summarizes research, be careful to accurately describe the research. Sometimes an attorney may ask you to change the language you use to summarize research, perhaps in the process subtly altering the meaning of the research. For example, when involved in a custody battle, your summary of the research about infants and mothers may describe important aspects of the "infant–caretaker" relationship. If the research is based only upon mother–child observations rather than both mother–child and father–child observations, then using the gender-neutral term "caretaker" rather than "mother" may be slightly misleading and should therefore be corrected.

Reports

The term "report" does not have a legal definition in the same way that an affidavit does. We are using "report" here to refer to any psychiatric, psychological, or social assessment prepared by a clinician for the purposes of a legal process. A report is different from an affidavit in that it is

---

[1]Many commonly used word processing programs have templates or standard format for legal documents, such as affidavits, that allow for numbered paragraphs or lines.

not a sworn or affirmed document. Tribunals may rely on information in a report if the information is not contested. If it is contested, then the author of the report may be required to provide oral testimony to prove the contents of the report. Even though reports are not sworn, they can be very persuasive to the parties and the tribunal. A good report is impartial, thorough, well documented, and consequently unimpeachable in cross-examination. If your report is particularly strong in these respects, the parties may feel better able to predict the results of adjudication and may well settle the case on their own. Accordingly, you can save a lot of blood, sweat and tears (including your own) if you do your best work up front, in the report.

The range of possible reports includes presentence reports in criminal hearings, investigation reports in child protection cases, custody assessments in divorce cases, parental fitness evaluations in cases involving termination of parental rights, assessments for juvenile transfer hearings, mental competence evaluations for involuntary committal hearings, and social policy reports submitted to legislative hearings. Some reports have few requirements for format and content. Other reports are regulated by statutes, regulations, or agency policies. Adoption laws, for instance, require the inclusion of certain information about adoptive parents in a home study, and adoption agencies have protocols for these reports that comply with the laws and expectations of the relevant tribunals. Clinicians can influence local guidelines by forming committees with attorneys, judges, or other tribunal members to develop better standards for specific types of reports if need be.

If Evelyn worked on an interdisciplinary team, how does the team decide which member should write the report? Reports should generally be written and signed by someone who qualifies as an expert. While a report could be restricted to fact evidence, most reports also include opinions. If Evelyn worked with a student who gathered some of the evidence, Evelyn may decide to submit the report under her name to give credibility to opinions in the report. However, if the primary reason for submitting the report were to document certain facts, then the student who gathered the information would be the most appropriate signatory.

Exhibits

Exhibits may include reports, affidavits, case records, photographs, clothes, and any other objects filed with a tribunal to become part of the tribunal's record of evidence. Exhibits are sometimes used to provide visual aids (e.g., charts or diagrams) to supplement written explanations in reports or affidavits. If an exhibit is introduced during your testimony, you may be asked to identify the object and how you are familiar with it. If a client left cocaine in your office and the cocaine was introduced into evidence, you would be asked whether you are familiar with this object, where you found it, who it belonged to, and how you know this. You may also be asked to attest to the chain of custody since you initially found it (e.g., if you gave it to the police). If you collect any objects that you believe may be used as evidence at a future hearing, maintain notes about how you obtained the evidence, keep it in secure custody to prevent tampering, and be sure you can trace possession of the object.

ELEMENTS OF REPORTS

The key elements of a report vary, depending on the nature of the legal and clinical/forensic issues, the requirements of the tribunal, and the contract between the expert and the party who hires the expert to produce the report (whether that be one of the disputants, the tribunal, or a public agency such as a probation office or a public advocacy group). The parameters of a report should be established before you conduct the assessment so that you can gear your investigation to the needs of the tribunal (see Chapter 7). The following subsections provide a comprehensive though not exhaustive list of topics that may be included in a report (Cameron, 1995; Catholic Children's Aid Society, 1993; Chisholm & McNaughton, 1990; Satterfield & Vayda, 1997).

Title of the Proceedings

If a legal case has been initiated, use the legal title of the case (e.g., *Philip Carvey v. Paula Carvey*). Identify the docket number[2] and the name of the court or other tribunal. If no case has been initiated, identify your report using the name of the party(ies) hiring you.

---

[2]"Docket number" refers to the number assigned by a court or other tribunal for purposes of identifying the case file.

Submitted By

Provide your name, address, and telephone number. Describe your agency and position. A brief description of your qualifications as an expert may also be included here. Often a *curriculum vitae* is attached as an appendix to the report.

Purpose

State the purpose of the report (e.g., an independent custody evaluation, a presentence report, an investigation into charges of discrimination). Identify the presenting legal issues as well as the party(ies) hiring you to prepare the report. If there is a court order or a consent order directing your work, cite the order and what the order says is the focus of your evaluative responsibilities. Briefly describe the circumstances surrounding the dispute.

Identifying Information

Identify the individual(s), families, or groups who are the focus of your report. Provide names, addresses, telephone numbers, relationships to the legal action, and relationships to one another (e.g., mother of Debra, Respondent in the action). For each individual, include the birth date, age, gender, birthplace, citizenship, and attorney acting on the individual's behalf.

Materials Reviewed

Provide a listing of all documents you reviewed while preparing the report. Include the name of the document, the date of its creation, to whom it was sent, and by whom it was sent. If the document is a court document, indicate the title of the document and its date of entry.

Positions of the Parties

State the original positions of the parties (e.g., Freida denies any professional misconduct; Paula is asking for sole custody).

Primer

Depending on the sophistication of the tribunal hearing the case, you may need to include a section designed to educate the tribunal about your area of expertise (e.g., the theoretical basis of your assessment; definitions of key concepts; information-gathering methodologies). Some reports need to be framed within the psychological or social variables that have been established in case law. When relying on case law precedents, cite the specific cases and include direct quotations explaining the psychological or social variables to be applied in your report.

Sources of Information

Identify the sources of data that informed your report. Identify dates, places, and people involved in any interviews. In addition to interviews, sources could include test results, file records, and other reports.

Relevant History

Family or individual histories should focus on information that is relevant to the current issues in dispute. For example, a presentence report should include information about past convictions. A refugee report should focus on the claimant's treatment in his country of origin.

Present Circumstances

Present circumstances could include a description of family dynamics, peer relationships, education, employment, and financial information, as well as other social, emotional, and physical data. Describe the subject's motivations and past attempts at change. Some reports require a broad psychosocial perspective. Others are focused on particular topics (e.g., a report on the current mental capacity of an individual). Provide balanced information, including both positive and negative elements. Use currently supported forensic methods and procedures in gathering information for the report (Austin, 2000; Gould, 1998; Gould & Bell, 2000; Gould & Stahl, 2000; Melton, Petrila, Poythress, & Slobogin,

1997). Ensure that you have included all of the facts that enabled you to arrive at your opinion.

Interpretation of Data

Describe the relevant data from the following sources as they apply to the case:

- Interviews with each party.
- Results from psychological test data.
- Information from collateral record review and interviews with collaterals.
- Direct behavioral observations (e.g., if the report is about issues related to parenting competencies, then you might describe your observations of how each parent interacted with the child and how you interpreted these behaviors).

Integration of Data

Discuss the degree to which information obtained from different sources of data converge or diverge on specific conclusions. Obviously, a specific conclusion is soundest when all data sources support that conclusion, while it becomes more suspect when one or more data sources support divergent conclusions.

Opinion

State your opinion or assessment of the individual and/or the larger situation, based on the facts provided earlier in your report. As noted in Chapter 7, opinions may include interpretations of data, expert assessments, and predictions of behavior or other social phenomena (e.g., the risk of a client committing suicide). Your opinions should be linked back to the stated purpose of the report.

Qualification of Opinion

Evaluate the factors considered in developing your opinion. Identify the strengths and limitations of the basis of your opinion (e.g., the reliability and validity of instruments used; assumptions made; support in the research literature). Indicate the degree of certainty with which you put your opinion forward. Use examples or analogies to illustrate complex points.

Offer rival, plausible alternative hypotheses. If you strongly believe in one interpretation of the data, then explain why you believe your interpretation is more strongly supported by the data than the alternative hypotheses.

Conclusions and Recommendations

Whether your recommendations are directed toward the tribunal or to the parties themselves should be negotiated when you are initially hired. State recommendations as suggestions rather than "orders" or decisions about what should happen. The parties and the tribunal can accept or reject whatever you suggest. Accordingly, it is important to provide a sound rationale for why your recommendations should be followed. Indicate whether one or both parties are willing to comply with your suggestions. If you recommend an involuntary option, consider whether your recommendations are within the tribunal's dispositional authority (e.g., some tribunals may not be able to order someone to undertake treatment). Offer alternative recommendations and provide the tribunal with your opinion of which recommendation(s) should be considered the most useful and why (i.e., the rationale for implementation of your suggestions).

Evaluative Summary

Highlight the key facts, opinions, and recommendations. In a presentence report, for example, include: the individual's motive for the crime; the precipitating factors; how the offense fit into the fabric of the subject's life; the individual's plans; and your recommendations for therapeutic intervention and sentencing.

Date and Signature

The report should include the date it was completed and the signature of the person who prepared the report. Updates and amendments should be prepared as separate documents.

Appendices

Your *curriculum vitae* and any other documents supporting your report may be attached as appendices. Depending on the nature of your assessment, you may also need to append copies of psychological tests or other key materials underlying your assessment.

PROOFING YOUR REPORT

Prepare and review your report with an eye to meeting both legal and professional clinical standards. In addition, be aware of the idiosyncratic expectations of your intended audiences. Check your report to ensure that it is readable, thorough, credible, impartial, and well documented. Use the questions in the accompanying Box as a checklist.

Checklist for Reports

- Is the language clear and concise?
- Is the level of language used appropriate given the sophistication of the tribunal?
- Have you gathered or shaped the facts in a way that supports a predetermined conclusion? If so, how can you conduct a more objective investigation and ensure that your conclusions are sound (unbiased)?
- Does anything in the report indicate bias (e.g., judgmental language, cultural insensitivity, lack of balance in fact finding)? If so, how can you paraphrase the report to ensure that it sounds fair and impartial?
- Does any of your information conflict with common sense? If so, have you adequately explained why "common sense" does not apply in this case?
- Does the description of the case provide sufficient factual background to inform decisions that need to be made?
- Does the report make any factual assumptions? Are there gaps in the information you have documented?
- Are facts, opinions, and recommendations clearly differentiated?

- Is there a logical connection between the facts, opinions, and recommendations? Is it explained in persuasive terms?
- Does the report include only information to which you can testify honestly, confidently, and knowledgeably?
- Are your opinions consistent with the research literature and with other reports? If not, have you provided adequate explanations?
- Is the format easy to follow through use of headings, numbered paragraphs, an index, or tabs for long reports?
- Does the report clearly relate to the legal issues in the case?[3]
- Are your charts, tables, or appendices easy to follow? Have you provided explanations for them?
- Does the report give an overall impression of professionalism (including spelling, grammar, format, and contents)?

Review a draft of your report with an experienced clinician or your attorney. Even the most highly regarded expert can benefit from having a report reviewed by a colleague.

THE USE OF LANGUAGE

Your close attention to language is just as important in providing written evidence as it is in oral evidence. In fact, written evidence can have even greater impact than oral evidence, since the tribunal sees it before hearing oral testimony. During deliberations, the tribunal may also look back at the documents after hearing the oral testimony.

As with oral testimony, use clear descriptive language rather than jargon, slang, or colloquialisms. Rather than use subjective terms such as "inappropriate behavior," give concrete examples of the behavior. Avoid equivocal phrases such as "it seems that" or "one may conclude." If the facts give rise to equivocal or contradictory conclusions, state them clearly. For example, "I observed X. This suggests either Y or Z. Y is more likely, because. . . . "

Check to see if any terms you are using have specific meanings in

---

[3]For example, a child protection report should not just provide an opinion about what a clean house is, but rather should connect this issue with the legal test for neglect.

law (e.g., informed consent, mental disorder). If so, make sure that you use these terms appropriately. Some clinicians use standard forms for reports or affidavits. The primary advantage of standard forms is that they use tried and tested clauses, based on precedent. For example, an affidavit in support of a welfare appeal would need to refer to certain standards established in welfare legislation. Having standard clauses for the affidavit, a clinician can ensure that the required information is included, even if the clinician is not an expert in welfare laws. Although standard forms can be an expedient alternative, the main disadvantage is that the clinician may be unaware of the specific connotations or consequences of the language used. Another potential problem is that the issues in some cases do not fit within standard forms. Standard forms must be updated to ensure conformity with changing laws. If you use standard forms, ensure that you understand the meanings of all of the clauses. Also, consider using the standard form as an outline rather than as a fixed format (see Appendix E for a sample affidavit).

Consider who may see the report. If the case settles privately, the parties and their attorneys may be the only ones with access to it. How will they interpret the report? If the case goes on to court or another form of public hearing, then information in the report may be widely accessible. Consider how you can frame the report in terms that are least embarrassing without losing the key information required by the parties and the tribunal. Finally, note the impact of the report on third parties. Will Debra have access to Evelyn's custody report now or when she grows older? Will one parent try to use the information in the report to turn Debra against the other parent?

The purpose of your affidavit or report is to inform, not inflame. Even though adjudications are adversarial by definition, the role of a witness can be carried out in a nonadversarial manner. Be humane, balanced, and sensitive. Use language that is direct but has the least stigma attached. For instance, suggest referring a client for a mental health assessment rather than for a personality disorder assessment. Your choice of words can have a strong impact on the overall tone of the document and how it is received. A report stating that "Philip was disturbed" could be rephrased as "Philip was upset." Similarly, "Paula refused services" could be changed to "Paula declined service." Consider whether your document helps or hinders chances for an amicable settlement. If you are a clinician in a treatment role who has provided a clinical report and testimony, consider how your report may affect your ongoing relationship with the client. Take your report seriously. Your recommendations can have serious consequences for the parties. Your words can also have a lasting emotional impact on the parties, regardless of the tribunal's decision. Finally, when you are preparing for a hearing, review the report with your client and help the client process his or her feelings about its contents (covered more fully in Chapter 4).

Chapter 9

Claims against Clinicians

For the most part, when a clinician is involved in a case as a witness, the clinician does not have a personal interest in the dispute. The dispute concerns a client or others who have a relationship with the client. The clinician may represent an agency, such as victim services or child protection, or a human rights agency. A victims services worker, for example, has a strong interest in supporting the needs and wishes of clients who have suffered from criminal offenses against them. Likewise, a human rights investigator is interested in identifying and remedying human rights violations. Still, the clinician's interests are based on a professional relationship. This chapter highlights the special concerns for clinicians as witnesses in situations involving their own potential malpractice.

Broadly speaking, a clinician commits malpractice when she causes harm to a client through improper performance of duties (Barker & Branson, 1993). How "improper" is defined depends upon the profession, how it is regulated, and the type of legal recourse that the client pursues. The criminal justice system is able to impose the most severe penalties, including fines and incarceration. "Improper" conduct in criminal law is defined primarily by offenses established under the federal or state criminal law statutes. Relatively few cases of misconduct by professionals amount to criminal offenses. Sexual assault, misappropriation of client funds (fraud), and unlawful confinement are among the most likely situations in which clinicians might be involved.[1] The primary avenues of legal recourse against clinicians are court actions and disciplinary hearings conducted by the clinician's regulatory association.[2]

COURT ACTIONS

Civil lawsuits can be initiated for breach of contract for services, intentionally violating a client's rights, or negligence. Negligence is the most common form of court action against clinicians. To establish negligence, the client must prove that the clinician owed the client a duty of care, the clinician breached that duty, and the client suffered damages caused by the breach. In most cases the issue of a clinician owing a duty of care is easily established. By simply offering or advertising therapeutic services to a client, the clinician is holding himself out to be someone who can help the client. Other issues are more likely to be contentious.

Different types of clinicians will be held to different standards of care.[3] Michael, who works as a mediator, is expected to live up to the standards of a reasonable mediator. Mediators are expected to respect a client's right to confidentiality. If Michael disclosed the Carveys' domestic problems to Philip's employer without the Carveys' permission, Michael would be in breach of his duty to the Carveys. If Philip lost his job because of this breach, then Philip could sue Michael for damages (monetary compensation for the losses or injuries he incurred). However, did Michael's disclosure actually cause Philip to lose his job? As a family therapist, Freida is expected to live up to the standards of "a reasonable family therapist." Consider the fact that the Carveys separated even though Freida offered to help them, utilizing a somewhat unortho-

---

[1]These offenses often include clinicians who exploit vulnerable children, people with cognitive impairment, and the elderly, particularly in residential facilities such as nursing homes.

[2]Most client complaints against clinicians are dealt with informally, between the clinician and client, or through various mechanisms within an agency (e.g., complaints registered with supervisors; in-agency appeals processes). How you respond at an early stage often determines whether a complaint goes any further (as was explained more fully in Chapter 3).

[3]Courts can impose standards of care even in situations where no express or definite standards previously existed. In order to reduce uncertainty, professional associations try to develop generally accepted practices for their members. The difficulty is that clinical intervention is partially an art rather than an exact science.

dox form of intervention. What were Freida's professional responsibilities? Did she fail to meet the standards of her coprofessionals in dealing with this situation? Just because therapy was not successful does not mean that Freida was negligent.[4] Even if she was found negligent, was her negligence the cause of the Carveys' breakup? How would emotional and social damages be calculated?

When one is a defendant in a legal action, knowing the issues in contention is crucial for preparing to be a witness. Ask your attorney to explain the nature of the legal issues and the type of evidence that you can use to respond directly to these issues. Michael would not help himself if he focused his testimony on how he never intended to hurt Philip, since negligence does not depend on intent. If Philip gave Michael permission to speak with the employer, evidence to that effect would be crucial.

Another form of lawsuit to which some clinicians are susceptible is "unauthorized practice of law." To practice law a person must be a licensed attorney. The most common trouble spots for clinicians are providing legal advice and drafting legal documents (for example, if Michael drafted the Carveys' separation agreement and advised them of the benefits of signing). If you are helping a client with legal issues, it is important to know the lines between attorney and nonattorney functions. In addition, keep records that document what you did and did not do. If Paula asked Sam for legal advice, he should document the request and how he responded. If Sam referred Paula for legal advice and Paula refused, he should note this in Paula's file. If Paula later claims that Sam provided legal advice, Sam will have evidence documenting the information he provided and actions taken.

Some clinicians are concerned that a client could sue them for defamation based on statements made while acting as a witness. Defamation refers to untrue written or verbal statements that harm the reputation of another person. If you tell the truth on the stand, you are not liable for defamation. It is unlikely that you will be sued based on statements you make as a witness, as long as you act in good faith and without malice.

---

[4]Consider a case where the client threatens suicide. If a clinician makes a reasonable assessment and things still go wrong, the clinician has not been negligent. The court is more concerned about how the clinician made the decision rather than the specific consequences of the decision. How much time was put into making the decision? What theory or research was used to inform the decision? Clinicians constantly make judgment calls. They are not expected to be perfect.

DISCIPLINARY HEARINGS

The various clinical professions have different mechanisms for dealing with client complaints. At one end of the spectrum, some regulatory bodies have mandatory adjudicative hearings with broad powers of discipline (e.g., suspensions, barring practice or compensation). Other professions have less formal dispute resolution processes, more akin to mediation or arbitration (see Chapter 10). Some professions may not require a license or certification to practice, so enforcement of participation in disciplinary hearings is tenuous. Many clinicians are not associated with any regulatory body, and clients in that case have no recourse for professional discipline other than what is offered in court. Because of the high cost of participating in court processes, disciplinary hearings are more accessible for most clients.

Some clinical professions have their own codes of ethics and standards of professional conduct. These codes establish the line between proper and improper practice. Conduct that amounts to a criminal offense or civil cause of action generally falls within the purview of professional misconduct as well. Professional misconduct also includes activities not actionable in court. Some professions, for example, prohibit a clinician from engaging in sexual activities with a client. Even though the state generally stays out of the bedrooms of consenting adults, these professions believe that such a rule is required in order to protect clients from clinicians who may take advantage of clients' vulnerabilities and trust. What if Freida's unorthodox intervention with the Carveys included surrogate sex therapy? If Freida were a member of a profession that prohibited sex with clients, she would be guilty of professional misconduct, even though other professions might allow it.

Issues often dealt with in disciplinary hearings include: role boundary violations (Reamer, in press); inadvertent disclosure of confidential information; diagnostic errors; inappropriate child placement; abandoning a client; premature termination without appropriate referrals for follow-up; defamation; failure to protect a client or third party from harm; and using a treatment approach that is inconsistent with practice standards and evaluative research (Reamer, 1995). A clinician who inadequately prepares to present as an expert witness could also be liable for malpractice. This does not mean the expert guarantees her client will win the case. The expert must carry out her role according to the standards established by her profession. Evelyn could be subject to malpractice claims if she did not verify information used to support her assessment or allowed bias to interfere with an assessment. Experts must produce fair reports, regardless of which party hires them. Experts can express strong opinions, but they may be subject to professional discipline if they state conclusions without having a factual basis or without considering alternative theories (American Psychological Association, 1995).

If a client complains to a licensing board, it is inappropriate to contact the client directly. There are two alternatives on how to proceed. The first is to respond to the licensing board with your explanation of the alleged issue. The second alternative is to contact an attorney and, together with the attorney, formulate a response to the complaint, with your attorney having all contact with the licensing board.

It is important to understand that the function of a licensing board is to protect the public. It is not to protect you. The board wants to maintain the public confidence that it is interested in and responsible for the proper examination of all legitimate complaints. You should take all complaints from a licensing board *very* seriously. No matter how you view the allegation, the licensing board will take all aspects of the allegation seriously. Remember that some members of licensing boards may not have expertise in your particular area of practice. They may need to be educated about aspects of your work and/or case law precedents that support your position. This is another reason to obtain counsel. Your counsel may guide you toward legal avenues of response that are unknown to you.

AVOIDING MALPRACTICE ACTIONS

The best advice on how to deal with a malpractice suit is to avoid it. From the client's perspective, he perceives that he has been wronged—and he may be right. From your perspective, you want to practice competently, do good for your clients, and avoid harm. A legal action is costly, time-consuming, stressful, and harmful to one's professional reputation—even if you *win* the action. A malpractice action is not all bad. An action is a means of ensuring that your practice is accountable. If you believe in a client's rights to competent clinicians, there needs to be a system of checks and balances. If you are sued, you can look upon the claim as an opportunity to work out a problem identified by a dissatisfied client. Most suits are settled before trial. If you are well prepared, even the court experience can be positive for you and your client. That said, you still want to avoid malpractice actions.

Even a competent practitioner who performs in a manner consistent with the standards of his profession can be sued for malpractice. Clinicians often deal with difficult situations and dissatisfied clients. A negative outcome may not be the result of malpractice, but an unhappy client may take action out of anger or frustration.

The tips for avoiding malpractice actions included in the accompanying Box are easy to list but difficult to incorporate into everyday practice. These tips will also help you as a witness if a malpractice action against you should arise. If you have acted competently, ethically, and judiciously, you will have strong facts behind you. You will have a much easier time testifying, since good facts make good evidence.

Avoiding Malpractice

- Ensure that you have the proper education, experience, and supervision for the type of clinical practice in which you are engaged.
- Stay within your area of expertise.
- Keep up to date with theory, research, and ethical standards in your field.
- Maintain timely, accurate, and thorough records.[5]
- Have the client sign a consent form that discloses the type of treatment, explains client and clinician roles and responsibilities, and describes the limits of confidentiality.
- When clients raise a complaint, respond empathically.
- Know when to call an attorney, your professional association,[6] or a colleague for assistance with ethical and legal issues, and do not be embarrassed to ask for help.
- If an allegation is true, consider admitting fault and offering an appropriate remedy; depending on the severity of the issues, legal advice may be warranted first.
- Be particularly cautious with clients who have a proclivity for bringing legal actions (e.g., people with paranoia, competitive personalities, or a history of involvement in courts).[7]

---

[5]Since malpractice can include actions *not* taken, be sure to document actions you considered but did not pursue. Be prepared to explain the rationale not only for what you did but also for what you decided *not* to do.

[6]Some professional associations allow members to ask for advice on a confidential basis, particularly with respect to how to deal with ethical issues.

[7]Some clinicians, concerned about allegations of sexual impropriety, avoid being alone with certain clients (e.g., by keeping a door open or having another person present).

TESTIFYING

Whenever you are part of a legal proceeding, consider whether your conduct can be called into question. What is the purpose of the proceeding? What is the role of your evidence within it? Find out if you or your agency is being investigated. If Evelyn were to be involved in an inquiry into a child's death, she should find out if the inquiry could lead to criminal charges. Some tribunals are only allowed to offer recommendations. In rare situations witnesses can be granted immunity from prosecution. In other cases your testimony at an inquiry can be brought directly into charges against you. Although this section deals primarily with testifying when there are specific actions against you, the information also applies to cases where there is just potential for future actions.

Are there any case law or statutory privileges that prevent you from being compelled to be a witness? If a client initiates an action against you, the client cannot claim privilege to prevent you from testifying for your own defense. However, if a nonclient makes a claim, you may not be able to reveal any confidential information about clients. Some clinicians have legislative protection against lawsuits. Child protection legislation typically protects Sam from being sued for professional negligence, so long as he does not act out of malice.

Ensure that you have legal advice to guide you through the process. Although some disciplinary processes do not permit legal representation at a hearing, you can consult an attorney before the hearing or have your attorney try to negotiate a solution. Ask your attorney to explain options on how to proceed, as well as their advantages and disadvantages. Find out whether allegations against you mean that you need to alter your practice until the legal issues are resolved. Suggest the names of other clinicians who could be used to support your practices and ethical choices. Review the suggestions in Chapters 4 and 5 regarding preparation and oral testimony.

Since malpractice claims are challenges to your professionalism, presenting in a professional manner is particularly crucial. Be conscious of your dress, mannerisms, and choice of words. Tailor your language to the composition of the tribunal, whether it consists of coprofessionals or nonclinicians. Ensure that your notes and records are in good order. If the case is based on claims of ethical misconduct, ensure that you are intimately familiar with the code of ethics for your profession. If the case is based on negligence, read up on the current standards of care in your field. Finally, avoid defensive responses. This is particularly difficult since your conduct is the focus of the allegations. Remember that your assessments and interventions are being challenged, not your whole being. Focus responses on your thoughts and behaviors rather than defending yourself as a person.

COSTS OF A DEFENSE

The costs of defending an action may be paid from a number of sources: out of your own pocket; from your agency or its insurance company; or from your own professional liability insurance. Malpractice insurance generally covers the cost of lawsuits for unintentional acts. Fraud, sexual assault, and defenses for criminal charges are generally not covered. Insurance policies vary significantly, and you do need to read the fine print to determine what is covered and what is not. Some professional associations offer assistance in terms of representation, information, and referral. They have an interest in protecting the reputation of the profession. Check with your agency, insurance company, and professional association to verify that you have proper coverage—*before* you get involved in any legal proceedings.

RESEARCH NEEDS

When clinicians are involved in research, few think of producing knowledge to be used specifically as evidence in malpractice cases. How do we know what the proper intervention is for a particular situation? How do we know whether there is a causal link between certain types of clinician misconduct and negative client outcomes? How do we assess emotional and social damages suffered by a client? As forensic specialties develop, perhaps there will be greater focus on malpractice issues.

The study of ethics has a rich body of literature that ranges from the abstract and philosophical to the concrete and practical (Corey, Corey, & Callanan, 2002; Loewenberg, Dolgoff, & Harrington, 2000). Most professions have a code of ethical conduct.[8] These codes vary in quality and continue to develop as new ethical challenges arise.

---

[8]For the code of ethics of the National Association of Social Workers, see http://www.cswe.org. For the code of ethics of the American Psychological Association, see http://www.apa.org.

In terms of legal research, there is considerable case law on malpractice. Case law is difficult to access for people without a background in law. Information in some legal journals is more accessible to non-attorneys. Some texts and journals are specifically designed for both attorneys and clinicians (McCloskey, Egeth, & McKenna, 1986; Parsons, 2000; Reamer, 2001; *Journal of Law and Social Work*). Still, much more could be done to narrow the gap between the professions, legal and nonlegal.

Chapter 10

Alternatives to Adjudication

While alternative dispute resolution has been growing in popularity since the 1970s, the role of witnesses in these processes has received relatively little attention in the literature.[1] In this chapter we deal with the role of witnesses in five types of alternatives to adjudicative processes: pretrial disclosures; pretrial settlement conferences; administrative tribunals; legislative hearings; and collaborative dispute resolution (including mediation).

PRETRIAL DISCLOSURES

Pretrial disclosure refers to processes where parties involved in a conflict are required to share certain types of information before the parties have a trial on the issues of the case. Pretrial disclosure ensures a safe and speedy trial. Since both parties know the case against them, they can prepare more effectively for the hearing. Surprise witnesses and testimony make for good cinema, but a trial is supposed to be a fair process, not an entertaining one. Pretrial disclosure often expedites settlement, because shar-

---

[1]The term "alternative" is a bit misleading in this context. The different types of dispute resolution processes are not mutually exclusive alternatives. They can be used in conjunction with one another, or in sequence.

ing information allows each party to assess the strength of its case. Even if the case does not settle, sharing information may settle some issues and enable the parties to stipulate to certain facts. Such agreement preempts the need to call witnesses to testify on these facts. Information obtained through disclosure can be raised at a subsequent hearing. A witness can be challenged and possibly his testimony discredited if information provided during pretrial disclosure is inconsistent with information provided at the trial. Disclosure processes vary among different types of cases and jurisdictions. The two basic types of disclosure processes are discovery of documents and oral examination for discovery.

Discovery of Documents

Discovery of documents generally occurs before oral disclosures, if any. The rules of the court require each party to provide a list of documents relevant to the issues in the case that are in the possession of the party or within the party's control.[2] The list may be supported by an affidavit swearing that all of the relevant documents have been listed. The other party can then request copies of the documents. If a clinician's evidence is relevant, these documents may include the clinician's notes, reports, videotapes, and computer records. Documents in the possession of a party's clinician are considered to be within the control of the party.

Some court proceedings require that each party specifically disclose the names of any experts to be called. They may also require that the party calling an expert provide a written report or statement summarizing the witness's credentials and intended testimony. If this information is not disclosed in advance, the party may be prohibited from calling the expert. Many states have statutory requirements or local rules for 14-day or 21-day or 30-day notice prior to trial.

The exchange of documents under discovery is the responsibility of the parties to the court action. Clinicians have little control over the process. If a client requests documents for discovery purposes, consider whether the documents are confidential or privileged (see Chapter 3). However, since a client generally has a right to his own records, clinicians need to honor a client's request for documents. If the client wants

---

[2]Applications for production of documents are also discussed in Chapter 3.

to claim privilege or challenge discovery of a clinician's records, then that is the responsibility of the client or her counsel.

The clinician's responsibility is in keeping good records on an ongoing basis. Knowing that your records may be requested during the discovery process, consider what type of information is important to include and how to frame it in a constructive manner (Chapter 6). If you are preparing a report as an expert witness, be aware that your report may be seen by the opposing party prior to trial (Chapter 8).

In order to decide which documents to make available to the other party, an attorney may ask you which documents might be relevant. If you leave out significant documents and the omission is later discovered, your credibility will likely be damaged. If you have lost certain documents, the attorney might ask how they became lost and where they are now. Are they in someone else's possession? Were they intentionally hidden? Were they destroyed? The examining attorney has plenty of room to try to cast suspicion on either your competence or your honesty.

Oral Disclosure

Oral examinations for discovery (or interrogatories) are question-and-answer sessions that take place prior to a trial.[3] Generally only parties named in the legal action or their witnesses can be examined for discovery. Oral discoveries, or depositions, are usually conducted in the private offices of an attorney, court reporter, or special examiner. Attorneys for each party are present in the room, along with one witness at a time. A special examiner may be present to oversee the proceedings, as well as a stenographer or technician to operate the video- or audio-recording equipment. Opposing parties may be present, but this is not necessary. The participants sit around a table. The witness swears or affirms to tell the truth. The opposing attorney asks the witness questions. The witness's attorney may interrupt periodically to advise the witness not to answer or to object to certain questions. The witness's attorney may also

---

[3]Some jurisdictions use written questions and answers. For each witness, the opposing attorney submits a list of questions. The witness provides answers in a written deposition, similar to an affidavit. While the contents of the answers are the responsibility of the witness, an attorney can assist with the specific wording of the depositions.

ask questions to clarify responses to the opposing attorney's questions. The amount of time can vary from a few minutes to several days (ask your attorney ahead of time for an estimate of the time required).

Some clinicians dislike disclosures because they do not want to breach client confidentiality or help the other side. If you understand the purpose of discoveries, you can see how they can be beneficial to both parties. Similar to discovery of documents, oral discoveries provide each party with an opportunity to be apprised of the other's case and avoid surprises at the hearing. Many cases settle following discovery. However, if the case goes on to trial, transcripts of oral discoveries can be entered into evidence at the trial. This is particularly useful if a party makes certain admissions of fact or guilt. If inconsistencies arise between what a witness says during discovery and what the person says at trial, the credibility of the witness's evidence will be called into question.

In preparing for a discovery, ask your attorney what information and documentation to bring as well as what types of questions you will be asked. Your primary responsibility in a discovery is to tell the truth, based on your knowledge, recollection, information, and belief. Do not try to use discoveries to present favorable information in order to win the case. The opposing attorney may only bring out one side of the case. The time for your attorney to argue her case is during the actual hearing. You do not need to disclose information other than that requested (White, 1994).

Most of our earlier suggestions for hearings also apply to oral discoveries: prepare by reviewing your notes and reports; use your anxiety management strategies; provide clear and concise responses; answer only what you are asked; watch for questions based on faulty assumptions; do not argue; do not try to evade questions; ask for clarification if needed; and do not guess at answers. Because discoveries are transcribed, avoid the use of gestures and vague utterances, such as "uh huh," to answer questions. If you lack firsthand knowledge of the information requested, state the information you have and its sources. Note that you cannot personally attest to its truth. "The psychologist provided me with these test results. I have no reason to disbelieve her, but I did not personally observe the administration of the tests."

Since the opposing attorney is interested in having you disclose information, the tone of a discovery is generally friendly or matter-of-fact. The attorney may use challenging or suggestive questions, but this is not a cross-examination, where the focus is on discrediting the witness. Questions tend to be detailed and dry. Neither the attorneys nor the witnesses show much emotion or dramatic performance. In spite of the differences, participation in a discovery can provide good experience for preparing for a trial.

There is no judge at a discovery to rule on the admissibility of questions (e.g., on the basis of relevance or privilege). The attorneys must work out any disputes on their own or take them to court, after the discovery. If your attorney directs you not to answer a question, follow her direction. Do not feel intimidated by an attorney who insists that you have to answer a question if your attorney advises otherwise.

For clinicians, one of the key areas of questioning is the source of information in client records and reports: what information did you observe directly; what information came from other professionals; what information are you inferring, guessing, hypothesizing, speculating, or assuming; and how have you verified your information. Some questions may be aimed at establishing bias (e.g., whether you like or dislike the client).

If there is information that you do not have available at the discovery but can obtain later, you and your attorney may be asked to provide an undertaking to give the information in writing. Be careful about giving undertakings on matters over which you lack complete control. Avoid absolutes. Instead, promise, "I will use my best efforts to obtain the following records. . . . "

After the discoveries, transcripts will be prepared. Review them for accuracy with your attorney. The other party has a right to be advised of any inaccuracies or omissions. This review can also save you the embarrassment of making inconsistent statements at trial.

Deposition questions tend to cover a wider range of topics than those permitted at trial. You should be prepared to answer these questions even if they may not be admissible at trial.

If you are an expert making a deposition, remember that the client's attorney is not your attorney. Consider consulting an attorney who represents you, either prior to the deposition or ask that the attorney attend the deposition with you.

PRETRIAL SETTLEMENT CONFERENCES

Following discoveries, but still before trial, many courts encourage settlement through pretrial conferences. These conferences are informal meetings between the parties, their attorneys, and the judge to try to resolve the dispute without the need for a full hearing. The attorneys for each party may be asked to provide an overview of the case. Witnesses are not present, and there is no formal presentation of evidence. Options for resolution are discussed. The judge may offer suggestions for settlement or indicate how he might decide certain issues, given the information presented at pretrial. If a trial is going to proceed, then the parties may be able to narrow the issues, streamline the process, and develop an agreed-upon statement of facts.

Although a clinician who is a potential witness does not take part in the pretrial conference itself, the clinician does have a role to play.[4] Prior to the conference, the clinician may be asked to write out the main points of her evidence for the attorney to take to the pretrial. If this information is clear, objective, and persuasive, it may facilitate a settlement.[5] Even if you are hired by one side, consider how you can frame your information in a manner that is constructive for everyone involved. Evelyn might be able to offer custody and access options that give both parents a legitimate role in Debra's upbringing. Sam could offer examples of Philip's parenting skills as well as concerns related to Debra's safety.

ADMINISTRATIVE TRIBUNALS

Whereas courts and other adjudicative tribunals are specifically designed to arbitrate disputes for conflicting parties, the functions of administrative tribunals—law making, policy development, law enforcing, and arbi-

---

[4]Some clinicians feel a lack of control, and even resentment, at being left out of pretrial processes, including settlement negotiations. If you have concerns about your role, discuss this with your attorney. You may be able to agree upon some type of role or sharing of information (e.g., helping the attorney prepare for a pretrial conference; participating in certain portions of discussions; receiving a brief of what went on at the conference).

[5]If your evidence is weak, that might also facilitate a settlement, but not in your favor.

trating—often overlap. The arbitrating role varies among tribunals, although there are similarities: interested parties have a right to notice of the hearing and a right to be heard. Some administrative tribunals use an adversarial process similar to that used by courts (outlined in Chapter 1). Others use a more investigative process. Rather than make the parties responsible for preparing and presenting testimony, the tribunal takes a more active role in gathering information and investigating the case. Members of a human rights tribunal may interview the complainant and the defendant in a discrimination case. A board that reviews the status of patients involuntarily committed for posing a risk to self or others will enlist its own experts to provide diagnoses and recommendations.

Clinicians can play a variety of functions in administrative processes, including fact witness, expert witness, advocate, client support, or tribunal member (especially for issues related to mental health and capacity). Clinicians may take on the role of client advocate if the tribunal does not require attorney advocates. The process and powers of an administrative tribunal are established by legislation, regulations, and internal policies. You need to understand the regulatory process in order to work effectively in these systems. Unfortunately, training for particular tribunals is hard to come by unless you work within the system (e.g., if you are an employee of a human rights commission or a member of a parole board). If you have no direct experience within the system, it is worth speaking with people who do. Explore the following aspects of the tribunal:

- Functions of the tribunal (decision making, policy development, enforcement).
- Roles of participants (tribunal members, disputants, experts, witnesses, advocates).
- Type of information on which the tribunal can rely (investigative processes generally do not have strict rules on admissibility of evidence).
- Types of information that will be persuasive (fact, expert opinion, political belief, values, emotional pleas).
- Manner of presentation of information (oral testimony, private interview, written).
- Names of other clinicians who have been involved in a similar administrative process.

Whether you are examined at a public hearing or interviewed privately, be prepared to answer questions as honestly, objectively, and fully as possible. As with adjudication, good records and reports will make your job as a witness much easier. Public court judges are usually generalists in the sense that they deal with a broad range of cases. In contrast, members of administrative tribunals deal with a narrow range of cases. The composition of the tribunal may include laypersons, experts, or a combination. The information you provide and the language you use to explain it should be geared to the level of expertise of tribunal members.

LEGISLATIVE HEARINGS

Legislative hearings are used by governments to gather information to make public policy and law reform decisions (e.g., on mental health, child protection, or criminal laws). Input may be sought from particular experts, interest groups, or the public at large. Clinicians often organize themselves to present information, deciding on a particular position and combining resources to provide a persuasive argument.

Acting as a witness for the purpose of influencing legislative decisions can be quite different from acting as a witness at an adjudication. In preparing for legislative hearings, consider their purpose, the history of the law, the current law, and proposals under consideration (Kleinkauf, 1981). For your specific hearing assess the type of information that will be most influential, whether it be professional expertise, anecdotal information (personal experiences of clients), political appeals, or positions with broad support (documented with petitions or letters; e.g., whether there is widespread support for allowing adoption by gay men and lesbians could be substantiated by an opinion poll conducted by an independent polling organization). Even if you are presenting as an advocate for a particular cause, objectivity is important to your credibility.

While truth and facts are important, decisions at legislative hearings are influenced largely by political factors. What goes on outside of the hearings is often more important than what goes on during them. That sort of advocacy goes beyond the scope of this volume.

COLLABORATIVE PROCESSES

Collaborative alternatives to adjudication include mediation, conciliation, family group conferences, and circle sentencing (in Native American communities). In each of these processes, a neutral third party
brings interested parties together to work out mutually agreeable solutions to their conflicts. The third party has no power to decide or impose solutions on the parties (Barsky, 2000; Mayer, 2000).

In some cases only the immediate parties involved in the conflict
are invited to participate in the process. Collaborative dispute resolution processes do not use "witnesses," at least not in the same way as
adjudicative processes. However, clinicians may be brought into these
processes in various roles. First, a clinician may be brought in as a support person for a client. In mediation, for example, Paula might be allowed to bring her clinician for moral support or to help her negotiate
with Philip. Second, a clinician could be asked to provide an assessment. Paula and Philip could agree that Evelyn would conduct a custody assessment.[6] Evelyn would then provide a report that they would
review in mediation. In preparing the report, Evelyn should consider
the same suggestions as discussed for reports for adjudicative processes
(as discussed in Chapter 8). In particular, the report should be written
in factual, balanced, and resolution-focused terms. Third, a clinician
could be asked to provide information from her previous work with the
client. For example, Philip and Paula may have a dispute about Debra's
parenting needs. Freida may have useful and objective information. If
the parties agree, this information could be brought into the mediation
process to help them make a more informed decision.

To be an effective participant in a collaborative dispute resolution
process, a clinician needs to understand how the process works. Collaborative processes focus parties on future plans rather than rehash-
ing the past and finding blame. Collaborative processes help parties
work together for win–win solutions. Collaborative processes encourage parties to keep an open mind about how to meet their needs and

---

[6]Before agreeing to conduct any type of forensic assessment without a court order, explore local state liability issues. In particular, find out whether you (as the evaluator) are covered by
immunity or limited immunity statutes when working outside of the court system. In some
states, such as Vermont, a clinician is not covered.

interests. If your clients are involved in such a process, you can support these efforts by the way you provide information and model for your clients.[7]

If you are asked to provide information for a collaborative process, find out if the information you provide can be used at a later trial.

---

[7]A fascinating new development is the collaborative law movement, where lawyers are trained to use nonadversarial negotiation processes to resolve their clients' disputes. You may wish to explore how clinicians can work within a collaborative law framework by contacting the American Bar Association at http://www.abanet.org.

Chapter 11

Conclusion

As clinicians and each of the clinical professions look to the future, more attention needs to be paid to the role of clinicians as witnesses. In the past, the legal profession has taken a leading role in designing formal dispute resolution systems in our society. Lawyers and judges have taken charge of how cases are processed.[1] They have decided when and how clinicians should be brought into these processes. While some clinicians have learned how to work within legal systems, most who have participated in legal proceedings have done so with little knowledge and even less control. In recent years clinicians have started to challenge traditional legal systems. Feminists and radical clinicians are among the strongest advocates for change. Other clinicians are striving to develop more equal partnerships with attorneys. Yet others have taken lead roles in developing mediation and other alternatives to traditional legal systems. Attorneys are also recognizing that dealing effectively with social conflict requires interdisciplinary collaboration. But where do we go from here?

One of the most effective ways to enhance attorney–clinician cooperation is to bring them together. Separate education, training, and practice tend to spawn ignorance and stereotypes about the other profession. Institutes of higher learning need to bring attorneys and clinicians together, whether it be through joint degree programs, joint courses, or joint projects (e.g., law students working in clinical settings or clinical students working in legal settings). In the area of continuing

---

[1]Judges, legislators, and court administrators also play key roles in how the legal system evolves and how cases are managed.

education, joint workshops and seminars would enhance interdisciplinary understanding. Interdisciplinary committees could be used to facilitate discussion and determine appropriate roles for attorneys and clinicians. In some jurisdictions, committees of judges, attorneys, and forensic clinicians have developed standards for gathering and producing evidence. Other clinicians, particularly unregulated ones, have had little input regarding their participation in legal processes. Higher standards of education, practice, and accountability may be necessary in order for these clinicians to gain influence. Clinicians from various disciplines need to work together, as past attempts to have certain mental health and related professions legally recognized have created divisions among clinicians.

On the research front, areas such as criminology, sexual deviance, mental disorders, and child abuse have received considerable attention. Unfortunately, relatively few counseling practitioners have been involved in developing research questions and designs. Greater participation from clinicians would produce direct benefits for clinicians as witnesses. A prime area for further research is a study of which factors contribute to a clinician's effectiveness in a particular type of hearing. While the reliability and validity of some diagnostic and assessment tools used by clinicians have been studied, many clinicians use tools that have little if any empirical support. There is also need for legal research to explore the relationship between scientific standards (validity, reliability, probability) and legal standards (admissibility, credibility, weight of evidence). Finally, research is needed to help identify the unique contributions that attorneys and clinicians can each make toward the resolution of social conflict.

Throughout this volume, we have emphasized the importance of conciseness. We will try to follow that advice in this conclusion. Our primary advice for clinicians as witnesses can be summed up in four words:

Prepare and be honest.

We trust that, by reading this book, you now have a better understanding of the roles that clinicians play as witnesses. While some of the information can be overwhelming, your newfound knowledge and confidence will help you to survive and thrive while participating in legal processes. Take what control you can. As for the rest, may luck and/or your higher power be with you.

Epilogue

You may be wondering whatever happened to the Carveys, their clinicians, and the other professionals involved in this case. Sam's child protection investigation determined that allegations of abuse against Philip
were unfounded. Both the child protection case and criminal charges
against Philip were dropped. Philip and Paula returned to Michael for
mediation. Emotional differences subsided when they began to discuss
the reason Paula threw Philip out of the house, namely, that Philip was
having an affair with their family therapist, Freida. Paula and Philip initiated a complaint against Freida through her professional association.
Evelyn and Michael were brought in as witnesses during Freida's disciplinary hearing and provided comprehensive, professional, and persuasive testimony. The tribunal revoked Freida's certificate to practice
family therapy. Philip and Paula agreed to a joint custody arrangement,
based on the recommendations in Evelyn's assessment. In spite of all of
the preparation, Lori was pleased that this case did not have to go to
court. Debra has grown up and is attending college, with plans to get a
joint degree in law and clinical social work. Freida gave up her family
therapy practice to pursue her lifelong ambition—to become an aero-
bics instructor.

Glossary

Adjudication. A process in which two or more parties present evidence and seek resolution of a conflict from an independent, third-party decision maker, such as a judge or arbitration panel.

Affidavit. A document containing information that is signed by a person who is swearing or attesting to the truth of its contents (see Appendix E for a sample).

Amicus curiae. Literally, a friend of the court (e.g., a clinician brought in under court order to provide an expert assessment; sometimes the *amicus* provides a brief written summary to provide the court with professional expertise on a topic relevant to the case).

Arbitration. An adjudicative process in which a private person or tribunal, rather than a publicly appointed judge, makes the decisions. Rules of arbitration may be governed by statute or agreed to by the parties.

Assessor. Used generically in this volume to describe a clinician who provides formal psychological or social assessments or psychiatric diagnoses (e.g., in vocational testing, custody assessments, DSM-IV-TR diagnoses).

Caveat. A caution or warning, often identifying a limitation in legal responsibility by the party declaring the caveat. For example, a clinician may assert that his model of intervention is effective but declare a caveat that he will not be legally responsible if the client does not follow certain specified instructions. A caveat may be provided to a client orally, but preferably it is in writing in order to ensure that there is evidence that the caveat was provided.

Circle sentencing. A process originally used in Native American communities to deal with people who have committed criminal offences. Various members of the community, including the offender, victim, family members, elders, and clinicians, are brought together to discuss appropriate remedies and to offer support. The process is designed to be healing-oriented as well as rehabilitative and deterrent of future crime.

Civil law. 1. Laws that regulate affairs among both individuals and groups, including family law, contract law, property law, child protection, and the law of torts (civil wrongs including negligence and malpractice). Although civil law primarily regulates the affairs between private parties, government agencies may also be parties to civil actions. Remedies for civil law tend to be compensatory, whereas remedies for criminal law tend to be punitive and deterring. Or 2. The type of legal system that operates in Quebec, Louisiana, and most of continental Europe, in contrast to the common law system in Britain and most North American jurisdictions.

Common law. 1. Law that develops from judicial opinions, principles, and precedents identified in cases tried in court (in contradistinction to statutes or laws passed by the government). Or 2. The system of law in most Canadian provinces and U.S. states (as opposed to civil law, which is used in Quebec, Louisiana, and most of continental Europe).

Compellable witness. A person who may be required by law to attend a hearing and provide testimony.

Consent order. A declaration by a judge reflecting agreement among the parties who consented to the order, in contrast to an order from the court that imposes a solution, whether or not the parties consented to the order.

Clinician. An individual who provides information, guidance, emotional support, or therapy to individuals, families, or groups; this designation includes psychiatrists, social workers, psychologists, clergy, and human service workers without professional education or status.

Criminal law. Law that deals with remedies for offenses against the state.

Cross-examination. A series of questions posed by an opposing attorney to challenge or discredit the witness's testimony or to bring out additional facts.

Defamation. An intentional tort, or civil cause of action, for making false statements that harm the reputation of another person. Defamatory statements made orally are sometimes referred to as slander. Defamatory statements made in writing are sometimes referred to as libel.

Defendant. The party against whom a claim, petition, or charge is brought. In some types of hearings, this party may be called the respondent. In criminal cases, this person is called the accused.

Direct evidence. Information provided orally to a hearing by a person who was a firsthand observer of the information being attested.

Direct examination. The initial round of testimony provided by a witness in response to questioning by the attorney who called the witness (conducted prior to cross-examination by the opposing attorney).

Disclaimer. A statement designed to limit legal liability by advising others not to rely upon certain information or not to use information for particular purposes.

Discovery. A pretrial process of sharing information between parties. Attorneys for each party ask the other party questions under oath. Questions and answers are recorded and may be used in the trial. Some jurisdictions allow for written interrogatories (questions) and depositions (answers by the witness).

Expert witness. A person with legally recognized specialized knowledge that allows that person to provide opinions based on evidence presented to the tribunal.

Evidence. Information that sheds light on the issues being tried.

Evidence-in-chief. *See* "Direct examination."

Fact witness. An individual called to testify about matters that the individual has directly seen, heard, or experienced. Unlike expert witnesses, fact witnesses are not allowed to provide opinions as part of their testimony.

Family group conferences. Meetings of family members and support persons, facilitated by a clinician. Family group conferences have been used primarily to help family members take responsibility for dealing with child protection issues or children who have been involved in criminal activity. Successful resolution within the family prevents the case from proceeding to court.

Forensic. Literally, of or belonging to courts or legal proceedings. Used in this volume to refer specifically to people from clinical professions who specialize in gathering and presenting evidence for use in legal proceedings.

Friendly attorney. Used colloquially in this volume to describe an attorney who does not represent the clinician but whose client's interests are consistent with the evidence and interests of the clinician. This is an attorney with whom the clinician will generally cooperate.

Incarceration. Confinement of a person convicted of a criminal offense, in a jail, prison, or other secure-custody setting.

Judicial notice. A rule of evidence that gives a judge discretion to accept commonly known information as fact without requiring the parties to prove the information by introducing evidence.

Jurisdiction. A geographic area such as a city, province, state, or country with a government empowered to pass laws over certain types of issues (e.g., each state in the United States regulates its own health care, child welfare, and licensing of professionals; in contrast the national government has primary jurisdiction over national defense and international commerce). Responsibility for criminal laws is split between state and national governments.

Legislation. Laws developed and declared in force by state or national governments (also called statutes or acts).

Limitations period. Length of time following a wrongful act in which a person can be sued or charged for that act; limits the period of time in which a claimant can initiate a legal action. There may be no limitations periods for the more serious charges in criminal law.

Malpractice. A wrongful act by a clinician or other professional in relation to performance of services. Legal recourse for malpractice generally depends upon proof that the professional breached a duty of care that was owed to a client and that the client suffered damages as a result.

Mediation. A collaborative dispute resolution process facilitated by an impartial third party who has no decision-making authority. The mediator helps participants come to their own agreement.

Motion. A request made to the hearing by one of the parties to the action concerning procedural issues or interim relief (decisions that affect the parties until the final decision in the trial is made).

Party. A social occasion usually associated with fun; however, used in this book to describe an individual, group, or institution involved in a dispute resolution process who has a direct stake in the outcome; one who brings a legal action or is named as a defendant in an action.

Plaintiff. The party who initiates a claim, petition, or charge; in various proceedings this party may alternatively be called the petitioner, claimant, appellant (in appeal cases) or prosecution (in criminal cases).

Privilege. A legal principle that may render information conveyed within a confidential relationship noncompellable in court. Although the attorney–client relationship is generally protected by privilege, privilege between clinicians and their clients cannot be assumed. It varies depending on the legal status of the clinician, the importance of the information to the hearing, and how the laws in each jurisdiction weigh the importance of protecting a particular type of professional relationship.

Pro se. An individual representing him- or herself, without legal counsel.

Res judicata. Literally, "the thing has been judged"; the legal principle that, once a matter has been decided in a hearing, the issue should not be raised again to be redecided. This principle forbids relitigation of the same issue.

Retainer. A contract with a professional (e.g., an attorney or clinician) establishing terms under which services will be provided and paid for; typically, the contract requires the client to advance specified funds to the professional prior to the services actually being rendered (see Appendix B for a sample agreement).

Sequestered. Detained in a protective setting during legal proceedings to prevent contact with others who may influence the detained individual by discussing the proceedings.

Standing. Recognition by a judge or tribunal that allows an individual or corporate entity to present arguments and information on its own behalf. If a witness is not a party to a proceeding, generally that person cannot provide information or arguments in an adjudication unless called as a witness by one of the parties or granted special standing.

Subpoena. A legally enforceable demand for an individual to testify in criminal court or to submit documents or other evidence. Failure to comply with a subpoena may result in a charge of contempt of court, which may be punishable by incarceration.

Testimony. Evidence given to a hearing by witnesses who provide information orally or in writing. In most jurisdictions a witness may swear to the truth of the information on the Bible or may make an affirmation.

Tort. A civil wrong, or category of legal action, where a party who suffered damages may sue another party for compensation or other remedies. Examples of torts include negligence, defamation, and nuisance (e.g., when noises or fumes emanating from one person's house disturbs a neighbor's enjoyment of his or her property).

Trial. A full hearing of the issues by a court or other decision maker that will result in a final decision on the issues being tried.

Tribunal. Used in this volume to refer to the decision makers in a legal dispute resolution process (including a single judge, a panel of judges, an arbitration board, a human rights commission, and other administrative or quasi-judicial decision-making bodies).

Undertaking. A promise to do something. For example, the attorney for one party may undertake (promise) to provide copies of the clinician's report to the other parties. Undertakings may be enforceable as contracts. Further, an attorney or clinician who gives an undertaking and fails to follow through on it may be subject to discipline by his or her professional association for breach of an ethical obligation.

Voir dire. The process of questioning a proposed witness to determine his or her qualifications (e.g., as an expert) or the admissibility of the proposed testimony. In jury trials, a *voir dire* may be held "in chambers" (i.e., the judge's private office).

Witness. A person who provides information to a hearing. In some processes, witnesses are required to swear to the truth of the information on the Bible or to make an affirmation of the information's truth.

Appendices

The appendices contain samples of the following documents:

A. Service Agreement for an Expert Witness for Review/Rebuttal Services
B. Fee Arrangement for an Expert Witness Who Is Called to Testify
C. Informed Consent to Participate in a Forensic Psychological Evaluation
D. Initial Letter to Attorneys after an Appointment Order
E. Sample Affidavit

These samples illustrate many of the issues that need to be covered in such documents. Still, each document needs to be tailored to particular cases, given the specific issues raised by the case and the local laws that apply to the case. To create your own forms and documents, consult with a local attorney who has expertise in the fields in which you will be testifying as a witness.

APPENDIX A. Service Agreement for an Expert Witness for Review/Rebuttal Services

The purpose of this Agreement is to explain the parameters of the role of [Name of Expert] as an expert witness for [Name of Client hiring the Expert] who is represented by [Name of Attorney], Attorney-at-Law, in the case between [List Names of Parties involved in the case and court reference number, if any].

[Expert] agrees to review a copy of the evaluation report filed in connection with the matter referenced above. [Expert] will review the text of the report and examine its methods and procedures, will review test data from psychological tests (if available), and will provide to the Attorney-Client an analysis of the report and of the evaluator's use of test data, conformity to current professional practice standards and guidelines, and use of forensic methods and procedures. [Expert] will provide opinions regarding both the strengths and deficiencies of the evaluator's work. There is no implicit understanding that [Expert]'s task is confined to identifying deficiencies.

If, on the basis of the information available, it appears that the evaluation was conducted appropriately and it appears that the conclusions drawn follow logically from the information considered, [Expert] will so inform the Attorney-Client either by verbal or written report. [Expert] will charge a fee for time expended and offer no additional services unless specifically agreed to in writing by [Expert] and the Attorney-Client.

If, in [Expert]'s view, significant methodological errors were made and/or the report contains significant flaws, [Expert] will consider amending his service agreement to include assisting the attorney in preparation for trial, to assist at trial, or offer expert testimony. If expert testimony is requested, [Expert] will prepare a written report to be used in [his/her] courtroom testimony.

[Expert] will *not* attempt to conduct a reevaluation. Because [Expert] is not conducting a comprehensive evaluation, it is understood that [Expert] will *not* offer an opinion concerning the comparative parenting competencies or custodial suitability of the parents. [Expert]'s testimony will focus on the analysis of the evaluation described above.

Fees for these services include a retainer in the amount of [Dollar Amount]. [Expert]'s work is billable at a rate of [Dollar Amount] per hour, and each hour worked is billed against the retainer. One-half of the retainer is nonrefundable. [Expert] will provide the Attorney-Client a statement of time billed on a monthly basis and at the termination of services. Should additional retainer fees be required, [Expert] will request these and the Attorney-Client will provide them in advance of [Expert]'s providing additional services.

Date [When agreement signed]: _____
Name of Attorney: _____ Signature: _____
Name of Expert: _____ Signature: _____

APPENDIX B. Fee Arrangement for an Expert Witness Who Is Called to Testify

The purpose of this Agreement is to explain the fee arrangements for [Name of Expert], who has been asked to testify as an expert witness by [Name of Attorney], Attorney-at-Law, who is representing [Name of Client] in the case between [list Names of Parties involved in the case and court reference number, if any].

Fees for the Expert's services will be billed at a rate of [Dollar Amount] per hour for Preparation Time prior to trial, and [Dollar Amount] per hour for Attendance Time. Preparation Time includes time expended while corresponding with the court, consulting with attorneys, preparing for trial, traveling to and from meetings with attorneys, and/or to and from court, and waiting (including any time that has been expended on this case prior to signing this agreement). [Expert] will record all interactions and provide a detailed account upon billing the Attorney-Client. Attendance time includes all time spent in relation to attending at the court, including time spent for going to and from court, waiting to testify, and providing testimony.

Fees for Preparation Time will be paid regardless of whether [Expert] is actually called to testify. If [Attorney] asks [Expert] to come to court, there will be a minimum charge for four hours of services [Dollar Amount], regardless of whether [Expert] provides testimony on that day.

[Expert] and [Attorney] acknowledge that [Attorney] has provided [Expert] with a Retainer of [Dollar Amount]. If, upon completion of [Expert]'s forensic services, monies are owed to [Attorney], [Expert] will refund the balance within 15 working days of the date of final billing.

If the trial is continued, settled out of court, or otherwise delayed, the Retainer will be fully refunded, less fees for Preparation Time, when notice is received at least five working days prior to the trial. Fifty percent of the "Retainer less fees for Preparation Time" will be refunded when notice is received at least two working days prior to the scheduled trial. Twenty percent of the "Retainer less fees for Preparation Time" will be refunded if notice is received less than two working days prior to trial.

If additional fees are charged, payment of outstanding fees will be paid within 30 days of the date of billing. If payment is not made within the specified time frame, [Expert] reserves the rights to charge interest at Prime Rate or to authorize the services of a collection agency or an attorney. All reasonable costs associated with their collection efforts shall be added to Attorney's bill.

All payments to [Expert] are for the provision of expert services as [identify professional background or expertise], and are NOT contingent upon providing particular opinions or upon a particular outcome of the case.

Date [When agreement signed]: _____
Name of Attorney: _____ Signature: _____
Name of Expert: _____ Signature: _____

233

APPENDIX C. Informed Consent to Participate in a Forensic Psychological Evaluation

The Role of the Evaluator

I [name of Evaluator] have been appointed by the Court to conduct an impartial forensic psychological evaluation. My purpose in conducting this evaluation is to gather information to enable me to formulate an opinion concerning what custody and/or visitation arrangement is most likely to be in the best psychological interests of your children. I may present this information to the Court or any other proceeding deemed necessary by the Court. Though the manner in which my fees will be paid has been determined by the Court, and though my fees are not paid by the Court, the work that I am doing will be done for the Court. Regardless of who pays an impartial evaluator, an impartial evaluator is expected to operate as though he or she was employed by the Court.

I do not presume that those whom I am evaluating are lying. However, I do not presume that they are telling the truth. Forensic psychologists are expected to secure verification of assertions made by those whom they are evaluating. Your cooperation will be expected as verification is sought of assertions made by you.

Confidentiality

Principles of confidentiality and privilege do not apply within the context of an assessment such as the one being conducted. Information provided by you, regardless of the form in which it has been provided or obtained, may be shared with others involved in the evaluation. Such information may include your statements, tape recordings, diaries, correspondence, photographs, observations outside the interview context, and other such materials.

By presenting information to others, verification of information provided can be sought and others can be afforded opportunities to respond to allegations that may have been made. Statements made by children may have to be cited in an evaluation report. It is important that you do not mislead your children. Do not tell them that what is said to me is confidential. It is not. Information concerning your payments for my services (amounts, sources of payments, form of payments) is also not confidential.

Office and clerical staff from my office who become involved in aspects of your evaluation are bound by the same rules of confidentiality and exceptions to confidentiality as I am under this consent form.

The need may arise for me to discuss the evaluation with other professionals and/or provide a copy of the final report to colleagues for their review and comments. In either case, all names and identifying information will be changed. In discussions with others who may assist in interviewing collateral sources, names are not changed.

Fees

Fees are determined through Court order or based upon an hourly rate of compensation. My hourly rate of compensation is [Dollar Amount]. Note that I reserve the right to increase fees with appropriate notice to you. Also note that fees for an assessment of this type are usually not reimbursable by health insurance.

A typical evaluation will cost between $4,000 and $6,000. In most cases, I will have expended some time prior to your receipt of this document. Fees are charged retroactively from the time that my services are initially requested and a file is opened. These fees do not include funds for work done after the evaluation is completed, such as additional correspondence, depositions, and/or trial preparation and testimony.

If, in my judgment, it is advisable that I consult with other mental health professionals, attorneys, or other professionals for purposes *other* than collateral information, time expended by me in such consultations will be billed to your account. I will not assume responsibility to pay for or forward bills for fees charged by other professionals who I consult for this evaluation. If another professional is consulted for the purpose of a collateral interview and it is their office policy to charge for such interview time, the cost of this professional's time will be passed on to the person(s) financially responsible for the cost of the evaluation.

Record-keeping requirements of forensic work make it necessary to log each telephone message and make a record of even the briefest telephone call. For this reason, there will be a minimum charge of [Dollar Amount] charged for any phone contact. All phone contacts will be charged at a prorated rate of [Dollar Amount] per hour.

Once an evaluation has been concluded, fees paid may be reapportioned according to the attorney's negotiation or the Court's direction. However, while the evaluation is in progress, I will not apportion fees based upon what was done and for whom. All work relating to the assessment is done in order to obtain as much relevant information as possible and cannot be viewed as work done for one party or for the other. Similarly, fees cannot be reapportioned in a manner that involves assigning financial responsibility for fees associated with other services to the other party (e.g., fees for a separate evaluation).

There may be times when an individual being evaluated will be required to pay fees for time expended by me in obtaining and reviewing information that the individual would have preferred that I not obtain or review. Similarly, there may be times when the financially responsible party (parties) will be required to pay fees in connection with the evaluation of a third party whom the financially responsible party (parties) would have preferred I not evaluate.

If it should become necessary for me to report allegations of abuse/neglect to the Department of Social Services (DSS),[1] the financially responsible party (parties) will be billed for any time expended in filing the report, being interviewed by DSS, and so on. This may mean that a financially responsible party will have to pay for time expended in reporting him or her to DSS.

There may be times when the actions of one party will make it necessary for me to make phone calls and/or write letters. In calculating fees for my services, no distinction is made between time expended in administrative matters and time expended in evaluation activities. Fees for time expended in administrative activities are apportioned in the same manner as other fees. This includes time expended in addressing fee-related matters.

It is to your advantage to organize any materials you submit for my consideration. You are paying for my time, and more time is required to review material if it has been poorly organized. Any items submitted to me should be clearly identified with your name. This is particularly important in the case of photographs, audiotapes, diary pages, and notes. Any item submitted for my consideration will not be returned. All items submitted for my consideration will be placed in my file.

The performance of evaluation-related services by me does not cease with the issuance of my report. Fees for all postevaluation services such as correspondence, phone time, attendance at conferences, review of court orders, etc. are the responsibility of the party requesting the services, unless other arrangements have been made. In the case of postevaluation services performed for the Court, it is assumed that fees will be paid by the financially responsible party (parties) identified in the Court order.

If I am called to testify at Court or to provide a deposition, you must pay for my preparation time and appearance. The scheduling of my testimony will be done in consultation with me and with appropriate recognition of possible conflicting personal and professional commitments. Your attorney(s) must provide me with notice of appearance indicating the approximate time of testimony. I will reserve this time for you and your attorney. I will not be on "standby." If you need my testimony, you will pay for either one-half day or one full day of my time. In this way, people toward whom I have other commitments will not be inconvenienced, as often happens in "standby" testimony. When you reserve my time, I am available to you at any or all of the time during that reserved time.

Limitations, Risks, and Services *Not* Provided

The profession of psychology has not developed specific methods and procedures for use in assessing comparative custodial fitness, and neither the profes-

---

[1]Different jurisdictions have different names for their child protection agencies.

sion of psychology nor the State of [Name of State] has established specific criteria. The criteria that I employ and the methods and procedures I utilize have been chosen by me and reflect, in my judgment, the current state of the art in conducting child custody evaluations. Any questions you have about these methods and procedures will be responded to during our initial evaluation session.

Please note that my report is only an advisory evaluation to the Court. The Court is not obliged to accept my recommendations. It is also possible, though not likely, that upon completion of a thorough examination of the issues, I may be unable to offer an opinion to the Court within a reasonable degree of psychological certainty. Fees for services already rendered will not be refunded under this circumstance or under circumstances in which completion of the evaluation becomes either impossible or unnecessary. If an evaluation has not begun, fees for time expended will be subtracted from any retainer and the balance will be refunded in a timely manner.

It is not possible to guarantee that an evaluation will be concluded by a specific date. Ordinarily, judges who have requested that forensic evaluations be performed wish to have the reports prepared prior to the commencement of trial. Though quite unlikely, a judge could begin a trial prior to receiving my report.

I will take reasonable steps to minimize the distress associated with the evaluation process. Nevertheless, though approximately 90 percent of the cases in which I am involved are resolved without judicial intervention, I must presume that there will be a trial and I will conduct myself accordingly. This means that information you provide will be questioned, and at times you may feel as though you are being interrogated rather than interviewed. In order to perform my Court-appointed function, I must be an examiner not a therapist.

I cannot provide psychological advice to an individual whom I am evaluating. If counseling or psychotherapy services are desired, please consult your attorney or other professionals for names of appropriate referrals. The pager used by my clinical partners and me is for emergencies of a *clinical*, not forensic, nature. The emergency number is *not* to be used at any time by anyone involved in a forensic evaluation. If you have an emergency, contact your attorney, physician, the police, the nearest hospital, or other appropriately trained professional.

Psychologists are admonished by our ethics code to release test data only to individuals qualified to interpret them. Unless otherwise instructed by the Court, test data will be released only to a mental health professional with appropriate credentials and training who is competent to interpret forensic test data. Additional information concerning this procedure will be provided to you and/or your attorney if requested.

If any questions arise of a legal nature, you must consult with your attorney. It is inappropriate for someone not trained in the law to attempt to offer an opinion concerning legal matters. I will provide no such opinions.

Psychological Testing

It is expected that when individuals being evaluated come to my office for the purpose of taking psychological tests, they will arrive unaccompanied. Spouses, children, companions, and friends can serve as sources of distraction. If someone must transport the test-taker, that person will be asked to leave and not return until the test-taker has completed all testing.

Submission and Retention of Documents

Your attorney will often be able to anticipate what documents an evaluator is likely to require. Obtaining pertinent documents prior to the beginning of the evaluation will expedite the evaluative process. Documents you wish me to consider must be delivered in a manner that ensures their safe transfer into my custody. Under no circumstances are litigants or others to make unannounced visits to my office in order to deliver documents. With the exception of certain test-related data, it is my obligation to produce at trial all items that I have considered in formulating my opinion. Therefore, my policy is to retain all documents and materials submitted for my consideration.

You are strongly encouraged to make copies of any materials you intend to provide to me. If you neglect to make copies and if you later require copies, you will be charged for time expended in copying these documents. If, prior to trial, a written request is made that I copy and release items in my file for examination by an attorney or by another mental health professional, you will be expected to pay the costs associated with producing these copies.

Out-of-Session Contact

Out-of-session contact between you and me should be avoided. It is to your *disadvantage* to communicate information to an evaluator in an informal manner. Limit your phone contact with me to scheduling appointments and addressing other procedural matters. I will not accept over the phone any information from you that I deem relevant to the evaluation.

Obtaining Information from Collateral Sources

Individuals being evaluated agree to authorize me to obtain any documents that I may wish to examine and to authorize communication between me and any individuals who, in my judgment, may have information bearing upon the subject of the assessment. In most cases, information needed from professionals will be obtained by telephonic interview as well as review of their written files. Individuals who are likely to be advocates for one party or the other will be expected to provide information in writing. I reserve the right to contact these people by phone for clarification and/or additional information. Some professionals may require you to sign a consent to release information to me.

I will be responsible for making all decisions regarding who must be evaluated, how extensively, and what information should be obtained and reviewed. There may be times when I will be asked to review information that I reasonably believe is likely to be more prejudicial than probative. There also may be instances in which I am asked to contact people whom I believe would be inappropriate to contact. I make the final decision about whether or not to pursue the information in such matters.

I reserve the right to consider any information regardless of the manner in which it has been obtained unless it has been obtained illegally. If I am asked to consider information that may have been obtained illegally, I will follow instructions from the attorneys if they are in agreement. If they cannot agree, I will request direction from the Court.

You may ask others to provide information about their direct observations of your parenting. It is your responsibility to explain to anyone from whom you solicit a letter that the information contained in the letter may be revealed to *any* of the individuals involved in the evaluation. This may include revealing information to your children in order to obtain their feedback and reaction. Your information or that of the collateral sources may be quoted in the evaluation report. Please ask each person to include his or her name, phone number, and address. I may wish to interview any or all of these people about their reported observations.

I will not accept any information via e-mail. I will not accept any information via fax unless it is from the attorneys or the Court.

Contact with Attorneys

Once I have been informed that I have been appointed to conduct an impartial evaluation for the Court, I endeavor to avoid *ex parte* communications with the attorneys representing the litigants. Once my report is complete and has been forwarded to the Court, I will engage in discussions with the attorneys as soon as they agree upon a format for that communication.

Allegations of Abuse/Neglect

I am required by law to report allegations of abuse or neglect. The penalties imposed on mandated reporters who fail to report such allegations are severe. If allegations are made, I will report them to the appropriate authorities, and my action in reporting them must not be interpreted as a display of support for the individual who has made the allegations. My action in reporting should also not be interpreted as an indication that I disapprove of the alleged actions of the person who has been accused. Most importantly, it must not be inferred that my reporting of such allegations suggests that I find them credible.

Postevaluative Developments

If significant time elapses between the issuance of my report and the date of the trial, I may request that the parties meet with me and/or undergo some type of follow-up investigation. If such a request is made, both parties must cooperate.

*   *   *

I ask that you thoroughly review this document and that you seek guidance from your attorney in the event that any aspect of this document is not clear to you. The evaluation will not proceed until both parties have expressed their understanding of and willingness to abide by the policies and procedures set forth in this document.

Your signature below indicates that (1) you have received, read, understood, and will abide by my evaluation and office policies and procedures; (2) you are waiving privilege with respect to any information in my file concerning this matter; and (3) you are authorizing the release by me of information, including my evaluation report, to the Court, attorneys, and other parties to which I have been directed to release the report by the Court.

_____	_____	_____
Client's Name	Client's Signature	Date Signed
_____	_____	_____
Client's Name	Client's Signature	Date Signed
_____	_____	_____
Evaluator's Name	Evaluator's Signature	Date Signed

Sign both copies of this form and return one copy to me. Retain the other copy so that you can refer to it during the course of the evaluation.

APPENDIX D. Initial Letter to Attorneys
after an Appointment Order

[Date]

1st Attorney's Name

Address

2nd Attorney's Name

Address

Dear [both attorneys' names]:

RE: [Names of Parties; Court Case Number]

I have received the [Date] court order signed by Judge [Name of Judge], in which I have been appointed to conduct a child custody evaluation. I have also received materials from both attorneys in the above-referenced case. Before we begin the evaluation process, please review the six enclosed forms with your clients before they call for their initial interview.

1. *Informed Consent for Clients* provides an explanation of the evaluation process.
2. *List of Collaterals* asks the parents to list the names and contact information of people they consider to be appropriate collateral sources of information for the evaluation.
3. *Informed Consent for Collaterals* is to be provided to each collateral source. Each collateral source needs to read, sign, and return the informed consent form to me with his or her written statement.
4. *Questionnaire for Collaterals* must be given to each collateral interview source identified by the parents.
5. *Statement of Understanding for Nonparty Participants* is to be used if either of the parents is repartnered and if either new partner will be asked to participate in the evaluation; it should be signed and forwarded to my office.
6. The *Parenting Questionnaire* (included as a paper copy as well as on disk in WordPerfect) must be completed by each parent and/or caretaker and returned to my office.

The initial interview may occur prior to each parent's completion of the parenting questionnaire. However, I need to have each parent's signature on the Informed Consent form when they attend their initial session. The retainer for the evaluation is [Dollar Amount]. Please forward the retainer, and upon receipt I will schedule the initial meetings with each parent.

Finally, I ask that the attorneys decide which documents, pleadings, and other materials will be necessary to forward to my office. I am particularly interested in any documents that help me to understand the legal issues involved in the case. I ask that each attorney copy the other side with all correspondence and materials forwarded to my office.

Thank you for your cooperation. I look forward to working with you on this evaluation.

Sincerely,

[Evaluator's name]

Encl.: Informed Consent for Clients, List of Collaterals, Informed Consent for Collaterals, Questionnaire for Collaterals, Statement of Understanding for Nonparty Participants, Parenting Questionnaire

APPENDIX E. Sample Affidavit

<u>AFFIDAVIT OF JONATHAN W. GOULD, PhD</u>

I, JONATHAN W. GOULD, PhD, hereby state and declare as follows:

1. I am a licensed psychologist in the States of North Carolina and Pennsylvania and am engaged in private practice in the areas of forensic and clinical psychology.

2. So that the court might be familiar with my qualifications, I offer the following brief background. My full current *curriculum vitae* is attached to this affidavit and incorporated herein by reference.

3. I received a bachelor's degree in science with a major in psychology from Union College in Schenectady, New York, in 1975; a master's degree with a combined specialization in clinical and school psychology as well as a Certification of Advanced Study in School Psychology from the State University of New York College at Plattsburgh in 1978; a PhD in Counseling Psychology from the State University of New York at Albany in 1985; and a Postdoctoral Certification of Training in Marriage, Family and Sex Therapy from the Marriage Council at the University of Pennsylvania School of Medicine in 1984. I am currently in private practice in Charlotte, North Carolina, and a principal in the private practice group Charlotte Psychotherapy and Consultation Group.

4. My primary areas of practice are forensic and clinical psychology. My forensic activities include, among other areas of forensic practice, aspects of child custody evaluations and assisting high-conflict, postdivorce families through the Mecklenburg County Parent Coordinator program. My clinical activities include working with parents and their children.

5. I conduct workshops on topics within forensic mental health, including conducting child custody evaluations and forensic ethics. I have also been an invited speaker at legal seminars on topics within the area of child custody, such as Keynote at the Los Angeles County Bar Association's Family Law Section's Child Custody Colloquium. I have presented continuing psychological education programs in child custody at meetings such as the Second International Conference of Child Custody and the Annual Conference of the Association of Family and Conciliation Courts. I have also presented continuing legal education at meetings such as the North Carolina State Bar Association's Family Law Specialization Conference.

6. I have authored a book on the topic of child custody, titled *Conducting Sci-*

entifically Crafted Child Custody Evaluations. I have written about child custody matters in national and international publications such as the *Juvenile and Family Court Journal* and *Family and Conciliation Courts Review.* I have actively participated in writing the revised Child Custody Guidelines for the North Carolina Psychological Association and am involved in several county family court subcommittees exploring how the Mecklenburg County District Court, attorneys, and mental health community can better serve divorcing parents.

7. I have conducted more than 100 child custody evaluations over a 15-year period. I have been qualified as an expert in forensic mental health, clinical psychology, and child custody.

8. My reason for detailing these aspects of my practice and training is to summarize my qualifications. In no way am I speaking in fact or by implication on behalf of any of the above organizations or institutions.

9. I have been retained as a forensic expert by counsel for the plaintiff, [Name of Plaintiff].

10. I have been asked to review the behavioral science literature pertaining to visitation arrangements for children under the age of 18 months and to discuss what types of visitation arrangements are generally recommended and why.

11. I have not evaluated the Plaintiff, the Defendant, or their minor children. I have not met any other interested party to this litigation outside of Plaintiff's counsel. I have not conducted a child custody evaluation or any other forensic evaluation of any party to this litigation. Because I have not conducted an examination of any party to this litigation or the minor children, I do not know if the conclusions drawn from the behavioral science literature review are applicable to the present situation. In order for a mental health professional to apply the conclusions drawn from the behavioral science literature to the *Baker v. Baker* case, a forensic evaluation of the parties and the child would need to be conducted. However, as guidance to the Plaintiff's attorneys and, potentially the Court, the educative purpose of this review may provide useful guidelines about current behavioral science research and literature pertaining to custody and visitation arrangements that generally serve the best psychological interests of a toddler.

12. *Normative development of infants and toddlers.* Children confront specific developmental challenges as they grow. Depending upon the age and stage of psychological development, the emotional tasks that confront the child will vary. Disruption in the opportunity to accomplish some of these tasks

may result in present and future deficiencies in psychological, psychosocial, and social functioning for that child (Whiteside, 1998).

13. In the first 12 months of life, infants accomplish an impressive number of developmental tasks. Their sleeping, waking, and eating cycles become regular and they learn varied and clear ways of communicating their needs. They begin to develop a view of the world that is organized, has object permanence, and has concepts of causality. They develop control over all parts of their bodies, learn that their actions can be goal-directed, and begin to anticipate future consequences. Most important in this process is the establishment of positive, smoothly functioning relationships with primary caregivers. Infants need regularity. They need to be picked up consistently when they seek contact. They need to be comforted when distressed. They require gentle caregiving. When consistent caregiving is disrupted, they can become difficult to soothe. Disruptions may appear in their eating and sleeping patterns. They may become delayed in language and gross motor development (Johnston & Campbell, 1988). Of particular concern is when the infant's relationship with the primary caregiver is disrupted (Main, 1997; Main & Hesse, 1990; Main & Solomon, 1990), especially in cases of marital conflict (Davies & Cummins, 1994; Owen & Cox, 1998).

14. The type of an infant's attachment to the primary caregiver is increasingly seen as among the most critical factors in fostering healthy development (Main, 1997). Infant attachment behavior develops slowly during the first year of life (Biringen, 1994). Although *parental* attachment to the infant may develop quickly after birth, the *child's* attachment to the primary caregiver develops slowly, taking typically 6 months or more to establish a preferential relationship to that caregiver (Main, 1997; Stroufe, 1983, 1991). Once a normative attachment to the primary caregiver is established, the infant uses the caregiver as a secure base from which to explore her environment (Ainsworth, 1982). Because the infant feels safe and secure in the context of the primary caregiver's presence, she is able to go some distance from the primary caregiver and explore freely. As distance from the primary caregiver increases, the infant becomes increasingly uncertain and fearful of her independence from the primary caregiver. This fearfulness activates her attachment behavioral system (Ainsworth, 1982; Bowlby, 1969), and the infant begins to seek out the primary caregiver once again. Activation of the attachment behavioral system may result from, among other situations, exploration of unfamiliar situations, exposure to unfamiliar caregivers, and care taking by nonprimary caregivers (Biringen, 1991).

I hereby declare under penalty of perjury of the laws of the State of North Carolina that the foregoing is true and correct to the best of my knowledge.

DATED [Date] at Charlotte, North Carolina.

_____

Jonathan W. Gould

Sworn to and subscribed before me on [Date]

_____

Signature of Notary Public (plus Stamp with Seal and Number)

_____

[Print or Stamp Name of Notary Public]

Personally known _____ or Produced ID _____ Type of ID _____

[attach list of citations and *curriculum vitae*]

References

Ackerman, M. J., & Ackerman, M. (1997). Child custody evaluation practices: A survey of experienced professionals (revisited). *Professional Psychology: Research and Practice, 28*(2), 137–145.

Amundson, J. K., Daya, R., & Gill, E. (2000). A minimalist approach to child custody evaluations. *American Journal of Forensic Psychology, 18*(3), 63–87.

Albert, R. (2000). *Law and social work practice: A legal systems approach* (2nd ed.). New York: Springer.

American Psychiatric Association. (2000). *Diagnostic and statistical manual of mental disorders—text revision.* Washington, DC: Author.

American Psychological Association. (1995). *Ethical principles of psychologists and code of conduct.* Washington, DC: Author. (Available online: www.apa.org/ethics/code.html)

Ashford, J. B., Macht, M. W., & Mylym, M. (1987). Advocacy by social workers in the public defender's office. *Social Work, 32,* 199–203.

Austin, W. G. (2000). Assessing credibility in allegations of marital violence in the high conflict custody case. *Family and Conciliation Courts Review, 38*(4), 462–477.

Austin, W. G. (2001). Partner violence and risk assessment in child custody evaluations. *Family Court Review, 39*(4), 483–496.

Austin, W. G. (2002). Guidelines for utilizing collateral sources of information in child custody evaluations. *Family Court Review, 40*(2), 177–184.

Barker, R. L., & Branson, D. M. (1993). *Forensic social work: Legal aspects of professional practice.* Binghamton, NY: Haworth.

Barsky, A. E. (2000). *Conflict resolution for the helping professions.* Belmont, CA: Wadsworth.

Ben-Porath, Y. S., Graham, J. R., Hall, G. C. N., Hirschman, R. D., & Zaragoza, M. S. (1995). *Forensic applications of the MMPI-2.* Newbury Park, CA: Sage.

Binder, D. A., Bergman, P., & Price, S. C. (1991). *Lawyers as counselors: A client-centered approach.* St. Paul, MN: West.

247

Bossy, J. (1985). *Disputes and settlements: Law and human relations in the west.* Cambridge, UK: Cambridge University Press.

Brodsky, S. L. (1991). *Testifying in court: Guidelines and maxims for the expert witness.* Washington, DC: American Psychological Association.

Brown, J. G., & Cox, C. R. (1998). *Report writing for criminal justice professionals.* Cincinnati, OH: Anderson.

Bruck, M., Ceci, S. J., & Francoeur, E. (1999). The accuracy of mother's memories of conversations with their preschool children. *Journal of Experimental Psychology: Applied, 5*(1), 89–106.

Cameron, D. M. (1995). *Preparing to be an expert witness.* [Video plus workbook]. Aurora, ON: Canada Law Book.

Catholic Children's Aid Society. (1993). *Legal services training manual.* Toronto: Author.

Ceci, S. J., & Bruck, M. (1993). The suggestibility of the child witness: A historical review and synthesis. *Psychological Bulletin, 113,* 403–439.

Ceci, S. J., & Bruck, M. (1995). *Jeopardy in the courtroom: A scientific analysis of children's testimony.* Washington, DC: American Psychological Association.

Ceci, S. J., & Bruck, M. (2000). What judges must insist on the electronically preserved recordings of child interviews. *Court Review, 37,* 10–12.

Cheatham v. Rogers. (1992). 824 S.W. 2d 231; 55 Texas Bar J. 1081 (12th Texas Court of Appeals).

Chisholm, B., & McNaughton, C. (1990). *Custody/access assessments: A practical guide for attorneys and assessors.* Toronto: Carswell.

Committee on Ethical Guidelines for Forensic Psychologists (CEGFP). (1991). Specialty guidelines for forensic psychologists. *Law and Human Behavior, 15,* 655–665. (Available online: http://www.abfp.com/downloadable/foren.pdf)

Corey, G., Corey, M. S., & Callanan, P. (2002). *Issues and ethics in the helping professions* (6th ed.). Belmont, CA: Wadsworth.

Corey, G. (2001). *Theory and practice of counseling and psychotherapy* (6th ed.). Pacific Grove, CA: Wadsworth.

Daubert v. Merell Dow Pharmaceuticals, Inc. (1993). 113 S. Ct. 2786.

Dickson, D. T. (1995). *Law in the health and human services.* New York: Free Press.

Faller, K. C., & Scarenecchia, S. (1998). *Testifying about child sexual abuse: A courtroom guide.* New York: Guilford Press.

Fradsham, A. A., & Lamoureux, H. (1995). *Presenting expert witnesses.* Toronto: Carswell.

Freeman, S. J. (2000). *Ethics: An introduction to philosophy and practice.* Belmont, CA: Wadsworth.

Frye v. United States. (1993). 293 F. 1013 (D.C. Cir.).

Fulghum, R. (1988). *All I really need to know I learned in kindergarten: Uncommon thoughts on common things.* New York: Villard Books.

Goldstein, R. L. (1988). Psychiatrists in the hot seat: Discrediting doctors by impeachment of their credibility. *Bulletin of the American Academy of Psychiatry Law. 16,* 225–234.

Gothard, S. (1989a, January). Power in the court: The social worker as an expert witness. *Social Work,* pp. 65–67.

Gothard, S. (1989b). Rules of testimony and evidence for social workers who appear as expert witnesses in the courts of law. *Journal of Independent Social Work, 3*(3), 7–15.

Gould, J. W. (1998). *Conducting scientifically crafted child custody evaluations.* Thousand Oaks, CA: Sage.

Gould, J. W. (1999a) A model for interdisciplinary collaboration in the development of psycholegal questions guiding court ordered child custody evaluations. *Family and Conciliation Courts Review, 37*(1), 64–73.

Gould, J. W. (1999b) Professional interdisciplinary collaboration and the development of psycholegal questions guiding court ordered child custody evaluations. *Juvenile and Family Court Journal, 50*(1), 43–52.

Gould, J. W., & Bell, L. C. (2000) Forensic methods and procedures applied to child custody evaluations: What judges need to know in determining a competent forensic work product. *Juvenile and Family Court Journal, 38*(2), 21–27.

Gould, J. W., & Greenberg, L. R. (2000). Merging paradigms: The marriage of clinical treatment with forensic thinking. *Newsletter of the Academy of Family Psychology, 3*(2), 3–7.

Gould, J. W., & Stahl. P. M. (2000). The art and science of child custody evaluations: Integrating clinical and mental health models. *Family and Conciliation Courts Review, 38*(3), 392–414.

Greenberg, L. R., & Gould, J. W. (2001). Merging paradigms: Clinical treatment in a forensic context. *Professional Psychology: Research and Practice, 32*(5), 469–478.

Greenberg, L. R., Gould, J. W., Gould-Saltman, D., & Stahl, P. M. (2001, Winter). Is the child's therapist part of the problem? What attorneys, judges, and mental health professionals need to know about court-related treatment for children. *Association of Family and Conciliation Courts–California Chapter Newsletter,* pp. 6–7, 24–29.

Greenberg, S., & Shuman, D. (1997). Irreconcilable conflict between therapeutic and forensic roles. *Professional Psychology: Research and Practice, 28,* 50–57.

Harris, J., Qualls, C. D., Harris, C. L., & Harris, D. G. (2000). Speech-Language Pathologist and interprofessional management of adult cognitive linguistic deficits. In E. Geva, A. E. Barsky, & F. Westernoff (Eds.), *Interprofessional practice with diverse populations: Cases in point* (pp. 29–46). Westport, CT: Greenwood.

Hunt, D. E. (1976). *Beginning with ourselves.* Cambridge, MA: Brookline Books.

Ivey, A., & Ivey, M. B. (1999). *Intentional interviewing and counseling: Facilitating client development in a multicultural society* (4th ed.). Belmont, CA: Wadsworth.

Kalichman, S. C. (2000). *Mandated reporting of suspected child abuse: Ethics, law, and policy* (2nd ed.). Washington, DC: American Psychological Association.

Kassin, S. M., Tubb, V. A., Hosch, H. M., & Memon, A. (2001). On the "general acceptance" of eyewitness testimony research: A new survey of the experts. *American Psychologist, 56,* 405–416.

Kirkland, K., & Kirkland, K. (2001). Frequency of child custody evaluation complaints to state psychology licensing boards: A survey of ASPPB member boards. *Professional Psychology: Research and Practice, 41*(2), 71–76.

Kleinkauf, C. (1981, July). A guide to giving legislative testimony. *Social Work*, pp. 297–303.

Krauss, D., & Sales, B. (1999). The problem of helpfulness in applying *Daubert* to expert testimony: Child custody determinations in family law as an exemplar. *Psychology, Public Policy, and Law, 5*(1), 78–99.

Lamb, M. E., Orbach, Y., Sternberg, K. J., Hershkowitz, I., & Horowitz, D. (2000). Accuracy of investigators' verbatim notes of their forensic interviews with alleged child abuse victims. *Law and Human Behavior, 24*(6), 699–708.

Landau, B., Wolfson, L., Landau, N., Bartoletti, M., & Mesbur, R. (2000). *Family mediation handbook*. Toronto: Carswell.

Lavin, M., & Sales, B. D. (1998). Moral justifications for limits on expert testimony. In S. J. Ceci & H. Hembrooke (Eds.), *Expert witnesses in child abuse cases: What can and should be said in court* (pp. 59–81). Washington, DC: American Psychological Association.

LeCompte, M. D., & Schensul, J. J. (1999). *Ethnographer's toolkit*. London: AltaMira.

Levinson, H. (1996). Giving psychological meaning to consultation: Consultant as storyteller. *Consulting Psychology Journal, 48*(1), 3–11.

Lilienfield, S. O., Wood, J. M., & Garb, H. N. (2000). The scientific status of projective techniques. *Psychological Science in the Public Interest, 1*, 27–66.

Loewenberg, F., Dolgoff, R., & Harrington, D. (2000). *Ethical decisions for social work practice* (6th ed.). Itasca, IL: Peacock.

Loftus, E., & Ketcham, K. (1991). *Witness for the defense: The accused, the eyewitness, and the expert who puts memory on trial*. New York: St. Martin's Press.

Luckton, R. C. (1978, November). Social policies, social services and the law. *Social Casework*, pp. 523–529.

Lynch, R. S., & Mitchell, J. (1995). Justice system advocacy: A must for NASW and the social work community. *Social Work, 40*, 9–11.

Madden, R. G. (1998). *Legal issues in social work, counseling and mental health: Guidelines for clinical practice in psychotherapy*. Thousand Oaks, CA: Sage.

Martindale, D. (2000, March 9). *Child custody and risk management*. Workshop presented at the American Academy of Forensic Psychology, New Orleans, LA.

Mayer, B. (2000). *The dynamics of conflict resolution: A practitioner's guide*. San Francisco: Jossey-Bass.

McCann, J. T., & Dyer, F. J. (1996). *Forensic assessment with the Millon Inventories*. New York: Guilford Press.

McCloskey, M., Egeth, H., & McKenna, J. (1986). Experimental psychologist in court: The ethics of expert testimony. *Law and Human Behavior, 10*, 1.

Melton, G. B., Petrila, J., Poythress, N. G., & Slobogin, C. (1997). *Psychological evaluations for the courts: A handbook for mental health professionals and lawyers* (2nd ed.). New York: Guilford Press.

Morgan, M. (1995). *How to interview sexual abuse victims: Including the use of anatomically correct dolls*. Newbury Park, CA: Sage.

Myers, J. E. B. (1993). Expert testimony regarding child sexual abuse. *Child Abuse and Neglect, 17*, 177–185.

Myers, J. E. B. (1998). *Legal issues in child abuse and neglect* (2nd ed.). Newbury Park, CA: Sage.

National Association of Social Workers (NASW). (2001). *Code of ethics*. (Available online: http://www.naswdc.org)

Orbach, Y., & Lamb, M. E. (2001). The relationship between within-interview contradictions and eliciting interviewer utterances. *Child Abuse and Neglect, 25*(3), 323–333.

Palmer, S. (1983, March–April). Authority: An essential part of practice. *Social Work*, pp. 122–126.

Parsons, R. D. (2000). *The ethics of professional practice*. Boston: Allyn & Bacon.

Paulo, M. A. (1987, May 9–13). *Expert witness: Before and during trial*. Materials from the Twentieth Annual Banff Refresher Course—Civil Litigation, Banff, AB.

Politi v. Tyler. (2000). 170 Vt. 428; 751 A2d. 788.

Poole, D. A., & Lamb, M. E. (1998). *Investigative interviews of children: A guide for helping professionals*. Washington, DC: American Psychological Association.

Pope, K. S., Butcher, J. N., & Seelen, J. (2000). *The MMPI, MMPI-2, and MMPI-A in court: A practical guide for expert witnesses and attorneys* (2nd ed.). Washington, DC: American Psychological Association.

Reamer, F. G. (1995). Malpractice claims against social workers: First facts. *Social Work, 40*, 595–601.

Reamer, F. G. (2001). *The social work ethics audit: A risk management tool*. Washington, DC: NASW Press.

Reamer, F. G. (in press). Boundary issues in social work: Managing dual relationships. *Social Work*.

Regina v. Carosella. (1997). 1 SCR 180. (Available online: http://www.lexum.umontreal.ca/csc-scc/en/index.html)

Regina v. O'Connor. (1995). 4 SCR 411. (Available online: http://www.lexum.umontreal.ca/csc-scc/en/index.html)

Saltzman, A., & Furman, D. M. (1999). *Law in social work practice* (2nd ed.). Chicago: Nelson-Hall.

Satterfield, M., & Vayda, E. (1997). *Law for social workers: A Canadian guide*. Toronto: Carswell.

Schetky, D. H., & Colbach, E. M. (1982). Countertransference on the witness stand: A flight from self? *Bulletin of the American Academy of Psychiatry Law. 10*, 115–121.

Schon, D. (1990). *Educating the reflective practitioner* (2nd ed.). San Francisco: Jossey-Bass.

Shuman, D., & Sales, B. (1998). The admissibility of expert testimony based upon clinical judgment and scientific research. *Psychology, Public Policy, and Law, 4*, 1226–1552.

State of Oregon v. Milbrant. (1988). 756 P 2d 620 (OR).

Sternberg, K. J., Lamb, M. E., Orbach, Y., Esplin, P. W., & Mitchell, S. (2001). Use of structured investigative protocol enhances young children's responses to free-recall prompts in the course of forensic interviews. *Journal of Applied Psychology, 86*(5), 997–1005.

Swenson, L. C. (1997). *Psychology and law for the helping professions* (2nd ed.). Belmont, CA: Wadsworth.

Tanay, E. (1978). The expert witness as teacher. *Bulletin of the American Academy of Psychiatry and the Law, 8*, 401–411.

Tarasoff v. Regents of University of California. (1976). 17 Cal. 3d 425, 551 P.2d 334 (Sup. Ct. 1976).

Wasyliw, O. E., Cavanaugh, J. L., & Rogers, R. (1985). Beyond the scientific limits of expert testimony. *Bulletin of the American Academy of Psychiatry Law. 13*, 147–157.

Watson, A. (1978). On the preparation and use of psychiatric expert testimony: Some suggestions in an ongoing controversy. *Bulletin of the American Academy of Psychiatry Law. 6*, 226–246

White, R. B. (1994). *How to be an effective discovery witness* [Video plus workbook]. Aurora, ON: Canada Law Book.

Woodbury, N. (1996). Pretrial interviewing: The search for truth in alleged child sexual abuse cases. *Family and Conciliation Courts Review. 34*, 140–168.

WEBSITES FOR LEGAL RESEARCH

American Bar Association: http://www.abanet.org

Megalaw: http://www.megalaw.com (includes links to statutes, court rules, and case law for each state)

United States Department of Justice: http://www.usdoj.gov

Westlaw: http://www.westlaw.com

Index

"n" indicates a note